Macrophages - Physiological and Pathological Hallmarks

Edited by Soraya Mezouar and Jean-Louis Mege

Published in London, United Kingdom

Macrophages - Physiological and Pathological Hallmarks
http://dx.doi.org/10.5772/intechopen.1009046
Edited by Soraya Mezouar and Jean-Louis Mege

Contributors
Changsheng He, Céline Rebours, Jean-Louis Mege, Jennifer Mildenberger, Jiexing Tan, Li Gong, Paulo R.Z. Antas, Soraya Mezouar, Teng Li, Yan Chen

First published in London, United Kingdom, 2026 by IntechOpen
IntechOpen is the global imprint of INTECHOPEN LIMITED, registered in England and Wales, registration number: 11086078, 167-169 Great Portland Street, London, W1W 5PF, United Kingdom

For EU product safety concerns: IN TECH d.o.o., Prolaz Marije Krucifikse Kozulić 3, 51000 Rijeka, Croatia, info@intechopen.com or visit our website at intechopen.com.

British Library Cataloguing-in-Publication Data
A catalogue record for this book is available from the British Library

Macrophages - Physiological and Pathological Hallmarks
Edited by Soraya Mezouar and Jean-Louis Mege
p. cm.
Print ISBN 978-1-83635-212-9
Online ISBN 978-1-83635-211-2
eBook (PDF) ISBN 978-1-83635-534-2

If disposing of this product, please recycle the paper responsibly.

Meet the editors

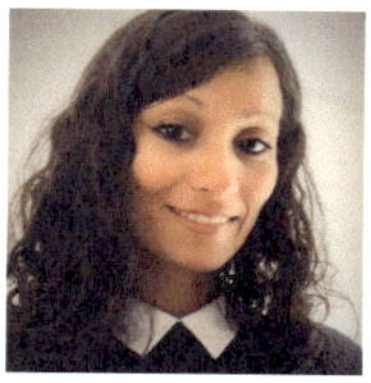

Soraya Mezouar is a Senior Researcher at the University of Aix-Marseille, specializing in the immune mechanisms involved in sterile and infectious inflammatory diseases. She defended her habilitation to supervise research in 2020, focusing on these mechanisms, and obtained her Ph.D. in 2015 on the role of platelets in inflammation, thrombosis, and cancer. His research focuses on the involvement of platelets in cancer and associated thrombosis, as well as the polarization of macrophages in infectious diseases such as COVID-19. She has published numerous papers in these fields and is a member of several scientific societies. She is also involved in training and scientific dissemination, supervising theses and coordinating master's degrees at Aix-Marseille University.

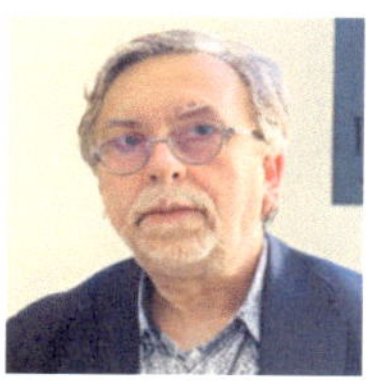

Jean-Louis Mege is a Professor and Researcher at Aix-Marseille University specializing in immunology and infectious diseases. He obtained his doctoral thesis in immunology in 1990 at the University of Aix-Marseille and was authorized to supervise research in 1992. He is also a hospital practitioner and has led research programs as well as training in human pathology. His work focuses on the biology of macrophages, intracellular pathogens, and the modulation of immune responses in infectious and inflammatory diseases. His publications include nearly 250 scientific articles in major international journals, addressing topics such as the intracellular survival of pathogenic bacteria, macrophage polarization, and immune biomarkers in infectious and obstetrical pathologies.

Contents

Preface

Macrophages occupy a central position within the immune system, at the intersection of defense, homeostasis, and tissue repair. Their remarkable plasticity enables them to adopt a variety of phenotypes, thereby responding to microenvironmental signals and contributing to both normal physiology and the pathogenesis of many diseases.

Macrophages – Physiological and Pathological Hallmarks provides an in-depth synthesis of current knowledge about these key cells. It highlights their multiple roles, from phagocytosis and antigenic presentation to the fine regulation of inflammation and tissue remodeling processes. By bringing together perspectives from cell biology, immunology, and experimental medicine, this book highlights the crucial role of macrophages as dynamic actors in maintaining biological balance.

This book is intended for researchers, clinicians, or students who wish to deepen their understanding of immune dynamics and the transitions between physiological and pathological states. Through this exploration, the reader will discover not only the functional diversity of macrophages but also their therapeutic potential, paving the way for new approaches in immunomodulation and personalized medicine.

Soraya Mezouar and Jean-Louis Mege
Aix-Marseille University,
Marseille, France

Section 1

Introduction

Chapter 1

Introductory Chapter: Macrophage – A Spatiotemporal Orchestrator of Tissue Rheostasis and Maladaptive Subversion

Soraya Mezouar and Jean-Louis Mege

1. Ontological diversity and the maintenance of the tissue niche

According to current macrophage biology, cellular identity is a developing feature of ontogenetic imprinting in conjunction with niche-instructive signaling [1]. According to current theories, yolk-sac and fetal liver progenitors produce successive embryonic waves that create tissue-resident macrophages [2]. These waves determine a foundational epigenetic landscape that goes beyond the conventional lineage versus environment dichotomy [3, 4]. Under homeostatic conditions, their strong capacity for self-renewal and longevity is controlled by a unique "ontogenetic memory" that is essentially independent of adult bone marrow hematopoiesis.

These embryonic lineages perform tasks that are essentially different from those of their transient, monocyte-derived counterparts and are crucial for extracellular matrix patterning and structural morphogenesis [3]. Therefore, the ability of these cells to maintain organ-specific rheostasis through a precisely calibrated oscillation between interstitial surveillance and reparative intervention while balancing real-time metabolic sensing with their ancestral developmental program is a defining characteristic [5]. The execution of essential physiological functions, particularly the preservation of tissue cleanliness and metabolic balance, is made possible by this ontological and developmental basis.

2. Physiological hallmarks: Efferocytosis and metabolic fitness

The macrophage's function as the major protector of tissue rheostasis, preserving local homeostasis by constant interstitial environment monitoring, further defines its physiological character. According to recent studies, macrophages are no longer passive scavengers but rather dynamic rheostat nodes.

Efferocytosis, which is crucial for stopping subsequent necrosis and the collapse of self-tolerance, lies at the heart of this stewardship. Efferocytosis, once thought to be the last stage of elimination, is now understood to be a highly instructional signaling event that actively reprograms the macrophage to maintain a resolutive phenotype [6]. This functional ability is inextricably linked to the bioenergetics of mitochondria. A “mitochondrial flick”, a quick response involving calcium absorption and dynamic fission, is triggered by the swallowing of apoptotic cargo, maximizing the cell’s ATP generation for successive engulfment cycles [7].

Beyond clearance, macrophages function as systemic metabolic sensors that integrate nutritional cues to regulate iron and lipid sequestration, protecting the tissue from lipotoxicity and oxidative damage [2]. In this context, metabolic stewardship is extremely spatiotemporal; macrophages act as “metabolic checkpoints” to protect organ function against fluctuating systemic demands by modifying their intracellular flux through glutaminolysis and the hexosamine biosynthesis pathway. However, when exposed to ongoing pathogenic stresses, the very plasticity that for such complex homeostatic care also makes macrophages susceptible to maladaptive reprogramming.

3. Pathological hallmarks: Epigenetic scarring and immune evasion

Recent research has focused on the critical function of macrophages across the spectrum of cancer and fibro-inflammatory illnesses, demonstrating their ability to control clinical outcomes by disrupting their homeostatic routines.

Persistent fibro-inflammatory states are caused by the “maladaptive reprogramming” of macrophages, in which fleeting inflammatory reactions fail to dissipate. By secreting ligands that encourage abnormal collagen deposition and myofibroblast activation, macrophages in chronic fibrosis undergo significant epigenetic remodeling that sustains a pro-fibrotic phenotype [2].

In the malignant environment, when macrophages are appropriated to redefine the immunological limits of the tumor, this failure of homeostatic resolution and the ensuing loss of niche fidelity are just as important as in organ fibrosis. Tumor-associated macrophages use their innate plasticity to adopt an immunosuppressive profile, thereby actively reducing T-cell-mediated anti-tumor immunity [8, 9]. This state is made worse by “metabolic competition,” in which macrophages eat local glucose and glutamine, depriving effector cells and encouraging tumor growth [10].

4. Concluding perspectives: Synthetic immunology and repolarization

The latest frontier in macrophage biology is reversing these harmful traits by synthetic engineering. The creation of chimeric antigen receptor macrophages (CAR-M), which enable the “re-education” of the immunosuppressive TME and the targeted phagocytosis of solid tumors, has enabled a major paradigm change in immunotherapy [11]. Understanding the spatiotemporal logic of macrophage activation would be necessary to develop precision treatments that restore homeostatic fidelity [12]. In conclusion, the macrophage’s dual role as a protector of tissue rheostasis and a catalyst for pathological divergence makes it the ideal target for both diagnosis and treatment in the upcoming generation of precision medicine.

Author details

Soraya Mezouar* and Jean-Louis Mege
Aix-Marseille University, Marseille, France

*Address all correspondence to: soraya.mezouar@univ-amu.fr

References

[1] Guilliams M, Bonnardel J, Haest B, Vanderborght B, Wagner C, Remmerie A, et al. Spatial proteogenomics reveals distinct and evolutionarily conserved hepatic macrophage niches. Cell. 2022;**185**:379-396.e38. DOI: 10.1016/j.cell.2021.12.018

[2] Nobs SP, Kopf M. Tissue-resident macrophages: Guardians of organ homeostasis. Trends in Immunology. 2021;**42**:495-507. DOI: 10.1016/j.it.2021.04.007

[3] Mass E, Nimmerjahn F, Kierdorf K, Schlitzer A. Tissue-specific macrophages: How they develop and choreograph tissue biology. Nature Reviews. Immunology. 2023;**23**:563-579. DOI: 10.1038/s41577-023-00848-y

[4] Musrati MA, De Baetselier P, Movahedi K, Van Ginderachter JA. Ontogeny, functions and reprogramming of Kupffer cells upon infectious disease. Frontiers in Immunology. 2023;**14**:1238452. DOI: 10.3389/fimmu.2023.1238452

[5] Blériot C, Chakarov S, Ginhoux F. Determinants of resident tissue macrophage identity and function. Immunity. 2020;**52**:957-970. DOI: 10.1016/j.immuni.2020.05.014

[6] Zhang S, Weinberg S, DeBerge M, Gainullina A, Schipma M, Kinchen JM, et al. Efferocytosis fuels requirements of fatty acid oxidation and the electron transport chain to polarize macrophages for tissue repair. Cell Metabolism. 2019;**29**:443-456.e5. DOI: 10.1016/j.cmet.2018.12.004

[7] Yurdagul A, Subramanian M, Wang X, Crown SB, Ilkayeva OR, Darville L, et al. Macrophage metabolism of apoptotic cell-derived arginine promotes continual efferocytosis and resolution of injury. Cell Metabolism. 2020;**31**:518-533.e10. DOI: 10.1016/j.cmet.2020.01.001

[8] Gomes Alves Martins R, Tekin MM, Cragg MS, Roghanian A. Therapeutic targeting of tumour-associated macrophage receptors. Immunotherapy Advances. 2024;**5**:ltaf009. DOI: 10.1093/immadv/ltaf009

[9] Mantovani A, Marchesi F, Malesci A, Laghi L, Allavena P. Tumour-associated macrophages as treatment targets in oncology. Nature Reviews. Clinical Oncology. 2017;**14**:399-416. DOI: 10.1038/nrclinonc.2016.217

[10] Reinfeld BI, Madden MZ, Wolf MM, Chytil A, Bader JE, Patterson AR, et al. Cell-programmed nutrient partitioning in the tumour microenvironment. Nature. 2021;**593**:282-288. DOI: 10.1038/s41586-021-03442-1

[11] Klichinsky M, Ruella M, Shestova O, Lu XM, Best A, Zeeman M, et al. Human chimeric antigen receptor macrophages for cancer immunotherapy. Nature Biotechnology. 2020;**38**:947-953. DOI: 10.1038/s41587-020-0462-y

[12] Shrestha S, Dick SA. Cardiac macrophages across space and time: Roles in homeostasis, disease, and remodeling. The Canadian Journal of Cardiology. 2026. DOI: 10.1016/j.cjca.2026.02.025 [In Press]

Section 2

Macrophages Generalities

Chapter 2

The Physiological and Pathological Characteristics of Macrophages

Yan Chen and Teng Li

Abstract

Macrophages, derived from monocytes, are multifunctional immune cells widely distributed in various tissues, playing crucial roles in both physiological functions and pathological processes within the body. They are integral to the immune defense of the body, participating in the detection and elimination of pathogens, the resolution of inflammation, and the maintenance of tissue homeostasis. This chapter provides an overview of the fundamental physiological characteristics of macrophages, including their origins, functions, and roles in immune responses. Furthermore, it delves into the modifications of macrophages in diverse pathological scenarios, encompassing inflammation, tumorigenesis, and autoimmune disorders. Recent research findings have uncovered the remarkable ability of macrophages to efficiently extract nutrients from dead bacteria, a process that could be harnessed for therapeutic applications. This chapter delves into the dual roles of macrophages in maintaining health and combating disease, emphasizing the significance of understanding their dynamic behaviors for innovative treatment strategies.

Keywords: macrophages, physiological characteristics, pathological changes, immune response, inflammation, tumors, autoimmune diseases

1. Introduction

Macrophages are multifunctional immune cells that originate from monocytes and are widely distributed across various tissues. They play pivotal roles in both physiological and pathological processes, being integral to the immune defense of the body. They participate in the detection and elimination of pathogens, the resolution of inflammation, and the maintenance of tissue homeostasis. In recent years, research has illuminated the complex dynamics of macrophage function, revealing that their roles can shift dramatically in response to environmental cues, leading to distinct phenotypic and functional states. This plasticity highlights their importance in health and disease, as dysregulated macrophage activity is implicated in a variety of conditions, including chronic inflammation, cancer, and cardiovascular diseases [1].

The physiological functions of macrophages extend beyond immune surveillance; they are also crucial in tissue repair and remodeling. Macrophages aid in wound healing processes by eliminating cellular debris and secreting growth factors essential for tissue regeneration. For instance, in the context of cardiac health, resident macrophages in the heart are crucial for angiogenesis, the removal of apoptotic cells, and the maintenance of cardiac function [2]. Studies have shown that these macrophages actively clear apoptotic cardiomyocytes through a process known as efferocytosis, which is essential for inflammation resolution and tissue repair. Additionally, macrophages contribute to cardiac repair after myocardial infarction by promoting the clearance and degradation of apoptotic cells, as evidenced by the identification of legumain (Lgmn) as a key mediator in this process. Furthermore, macrophages play a significant role in the heart's electrical conduction system, with their presence being vital for preventing fibrosis and stimulating angiogenesis, thereby maintaining cardiac function. However, when faced with pathological conditions, such as infection or injury, macrophages can adopt a pro-inflammatory M1 phenotype, which, if not properly regulated, can lead to excessive inflammation and subsequent tissue damage. This duality of function highlights the importance of understanding the regulatory mechanisms that govern macrophage behavior in various contexts [3].

Recent studies have also highlighted the role of macrophages in metabolic regulation, particularly in the context of obesity and metabolic syndrome. Adipose tissue macrophages (ATMs) have been shown to play a pivotal role in systemic metabolism by secreting pro-inflammatory cytokines, which contribute to insulin resistance and other metabolic disorders [4]. Studies have demonstrated that macrophage UBE2M is crucial for obesity-induced inflammation, and the molecular mechanism involving CD146 promotes inflammatory polarization of ATMs, further highlighting their impact on metabolic responses to obesity. The interplay between macrophages and metabolic pathways underscores their central role in linking immune responses with metabolic health, suggesting that targeting macrophage function could be a viable therapeutic strategy for metabolic diseases [5].

Furthermore, the pathological characteristics of macrophages have attracted considerable attention within the oncology field. Tumor-associated macrophages (TAMs) display a distinct phenotype that promotes tumor growth, invasion, and metastasis. These cells can establish an immunosuppressive microenvironment that aids in cancer progression and resistance to treatment [6]. Comprehending the mechanisms behind

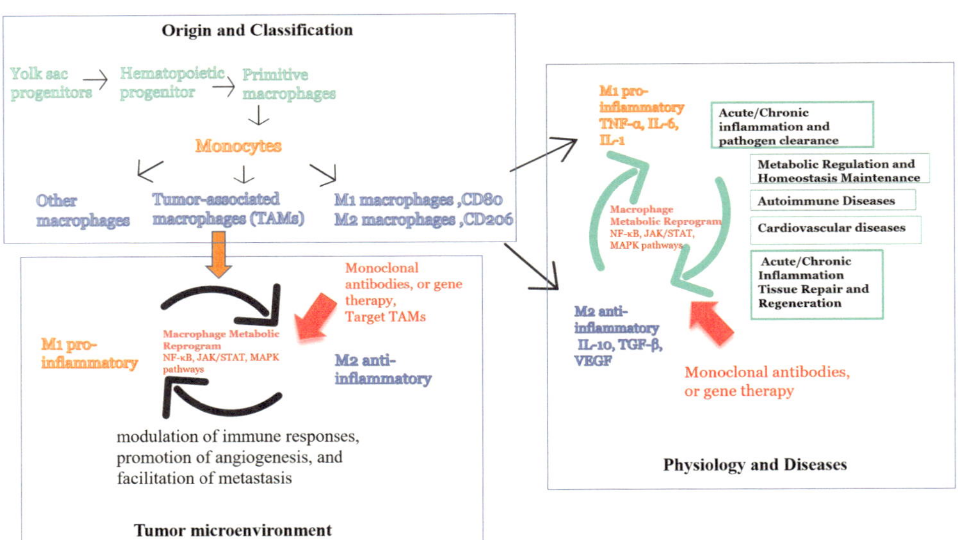

Figure 1.
The physiological and pathological role of macrophages.

macrophage polarization within tumors is essential for the development of effective immunotherapies that aim to reprogram TAMs into anti-tumor phenotypes [3].

In addition to their roles in cancer and metabolic diseases, macrophages are also critical players in the pathogenesis of autoimmune diseases and chronic inflammatory conditions. For instance, in rheumatoid arthritis, macrophages contribute to joint inflammation and damage by producing inflammatory mediators and interacting with other immune cells [7]. The complex interactions between macrophages and other cells within the immune system underscore the necessity for a comprehensive understanding of macrophage biology to inform therapeutic strategies aimed at modulating their activity in various disease states [8].

In summary, macrophages are essential components of the immune system, with diverse roles that span from immune defense to tissue repair and metabolic regulation. Their ability to adapt to various physiological and pathological environments makes them a focal point of research aimed at understanding disease mechanisms and developing targeted therapies. Continued exploration of macrophage biology is vital for uncovering new therapeutic opportunities that could improve outcomes in a range of diseases, from chronic inflammatory conditions to cancer (**Figure 1**) [9].

2. Main text

2.1 Macrophage origin and classification

2.1.1 Developmental process of macrophages

Macrophages originate from distinct hematopoietic progenitor cells during embryonic development and throughout life. Initially, they arise from yolk sac progenitors in the embryo, which give rise to primitive macrophages that populate various tissues. This early wave of macrophages is crucial for establishing tissue homeostasis and immune surveillance. As development progresses, definitive hematopoiesis occurs in the fetal liver and later in the bone marrow, leading to the generation of monocytes that migrate into tissues and differentiate into macrophages. This process is tightly regulated by various cytokines and transcription factors, such as colony-stimulating factor 1 (CSF1) and its receptor (CSF1R), which play vital roles in monocyte survival, proliferation, and differentiation into macrophages [6]. Recent studies have highlighted the plasticity of macrophages, demonstrating that they can adapt their phenotype and function in response to environmental cues, which is essential for their roles in both homeostasis and disease [1].

2.1.2 Classification and functions of macrophages

Macrophages can be broadly classified into two main categories based on their activation states: M1 (classically activated) and M2 (alternatively activated) macrophages. M1 macrophages are typically associated with pro-inflammatory responses, producing cytokines such as TNF-α and IL-6, and are crucial for combating infections and facilitating tissue damage repair. In contrast, M2 macrophages are linked to anti-inflammatory responses, promoting tissue repair and remodeling by secreting anti-inflammatory cytokines like IL-10 and TGF-β [10]. This classification, however, is an oversimplification, as macrophages exhibit a spectrum of functional phenotypes influenced by their microenvironment. For instance, tumor-associated macrophages

(TAMs) display a unique phenotype that supports tumor growth and metastasis, highlighting the importance of context in macrophage function [11]. Understanding the diverse roles of macrophages in various physiological and pathological conditions is crucial for developing targeted therapies aimed at modulating their activity in diseases such as cancer and chronic inflammatory disorders [12].

2.1.3 Phenotypic characteristics of macrophages

Macrophages display a remarkable degree of heterogeneity in their phenotypic characteristics, which can be evaluated using various markers and functional assays. Surface markers such as CD68, CD163, and MHC class II are commonly utilized to identify macrophage populations and their activation states. For instance, M1 macrophages typically express high levels of CD80 and low levels of CD206, whereas M2 macrophages exhibit the opposite pattern [6]. Furthermore, metabolic profiling has uncovered distinct metabolic pathways associated with different macrophage phenotypes, with M1 macrophages favoring glycolysis and M2 macrophages showing enhanced oxidative phosphorylation [13]. The plasticity of macrophages enables them to swiftly adapt to environmental changes, a crucial aspect of their roles in immune responses and tissue homeostasis. Recent advances in single-cell transcriptomics have further clarified the complexity of macrophage phenotypes, revealing subpopulations with unique transcriptional profiles that correspond to specific functional outcomes in health and disease [6]. This ongoing research highlights the necessity for a nuanced comprehension of macrophage biology to guide therapeutic strategies targeting these adaptable immune cells.

2.2 Macrophages in physiological processes

2.2.1 Immune surveillance and pathogen clearance

Macrophages play a pivotal role in immune surveillance, acting as the first line of defense against pathogens. They are equipped with various pattern recognition receptors (PRRs) that enable them to detect pathogen-associated molecular patterns (PAMPs) and danger-associated molecular patterns (DAMPs). Upon recognition, macrophages initiate pro-inflammatory responses by secreting cytokines and chemokines, which recruit additional immune cells to the site of infection. This process is crucial for the containment and elimination of pathogens. Furthermore, macrophages can polarize into distinct phenotypes, primarily M1 (pro-inflammatory) and M2 (anti-inflammatory), which dictate their functional outcomes. M1 macrophages are associated with the clearance of intracellular pathogens and the activation of T cells, while M2 macrophages facilitate tissue repair and resolution of inflammation. Recent studies have highlighted the importance of macrophage metabolism in modulating their immune functions, where metabolic reprogramming influences their polarization and effector functions during immune responses [1, 10]. This metabolic flexibility allows macrophages to adapt to varying microenvironments and maintain homeostasis while effectively responding to infections.

2.2.2 Tissue repair and regeneration

Macrophages play a crucial role in tissue repair and regeneration, in addition to their function in immune defense. Following injury, they are recruited to the damaged area where they manage the healing process through a series of well-coordinated actions. Macrophages clear apoptotic cells and debris *via* efferocytosis, a process essential for preventing chronic inflammation and promoting tissue regeneration. They also secrete various growth factors and cytokines, including transforming growth factor-beta (TGF-β) and vascular endothelial growth factor (VEGF), which are vital for angiogenesis and the recruitment of progenitor cells to the injury site [3, 9]. The balance between M1 and M2 macrophage polarization is critical during the healing process; M1 macrophages promote inflammation and pathogen clearance, whereas M2 macrophages facilitate tissue repair and remodeling. Dysregulation of macrophage function can result in impaired healing and chronic wounds, underscoring the importance of understanding macrophage biology to develop therapeutic strategies for enhancing tissue regeneration [14, 15].

2.2.3 Metabolic regulation and homeostasis maintenance

Macrophages are significant not only as immune cells but also in metabolic regulation and the maintenance of tissue homeostasis. They are involved in the regulation of energy metabolism, influencing processes such as glucose homeostasis and lipid metabolism. In adipose tissue, macrophages can adopt different phenotypes in response to the tissue's metabolic state. For example, in obesity, the accumulation of pro-inflammatory M1 macrophages contributes to insulin resistance and metabolic dysfunction, while M2 macrophages promote anti-inflammatory responses and tissue repair [5, 16]. The interaction between macrophages and other cell types, such as adipocytes and myocytes, is essential for maintaining metabolic balance. Furthermore, macrophages can impact systemic metabolism by secreting adipokines and cytokines, which can affect insulin sensitivity and energy expenditure. Understanding the metabolic functions of macrophages reveals new opportunities for therapeutic interventions in metabolic disorders, highlighting their role as key players in both immune and metabolic homeostasis [17, 18].

2.3 The role of macrophages in inflammation

2.3.1 Acute inflammatory response

Macrophages are essential players in the acute inflammatory response, serving as the first line of defense against pathogens and tissue injury. Upon detecting harmful stimuli, such as pathogens or damaged cells, macrophages rapidly migrate to the site of injury, where they perform several critical functions. They recognize pathogens through pattern recognition receptors (PRRs), which leads to the activation of pro-inflammatory signaling pathways. This, in turn, results in the production and release of cytokines and chemokines. These signaling molecules recruit additional immune cells, such as neutrophils, to the site of inflammation, amplifying the inflammatory response [19]. Furthermore, macrophages exhibit remarkable plasticity, allowing them to polarize into distinct phenotypes, primarily the M1 (pro-inflammatory) and M2 (anti-inflammatory) macrophages. M1 macrophages are characterized by their ability to produce pro-inflammatory cytokines such as TNF-α, IL-1β, and IL-6, which are crucial for pathogen clearance and the initiation of tissue repair processes [3]. However, the prolonged activation of M1 macrophages can lead to tissue damage and contribute to chronic inflammatory conditions if not properly regulated. Thus, the timely resolution of acute inflammation is vital, and macrophages play a pivotal role in this process by transitioning from a pro-inflammatory to an anti-inflammatory phenotype, facilitating tissue repair and homeostasis [20].

2.3.2 Chronic inflammation and its mechanisms

Chronic inflammation is characterized by the persistent activation of the immune response, often due to unresolved acute inflammation, autoimmune diseases, or chronic infections. In this context, macrophages undergo a shift in their functional phenotype, often becoming pro-inflammatory M1 macrophages that secrete a variety of inflammatory mediators, perpetuating the inflammatory cycle [21]. The mechanisms underlying this transition involve a complex interplay of signaling pathways, including the NF-κB and MAPK pathways, which are activated by various stimuli, including cytokines and pathogen-associated molecular patterns (PAMPs) [22]. Furthermore, the metabolic reprogramming of macrophages plays a crucial role in their polarization and function during chronic inflammation. For instance, the shift toward aerobic glycolysis in M1 macrophages supports their inflammatory functions, while M2 macrophages rely more on oxidative phosphorylation and fatty acid oxidation for their anti-inflammatory roles [20]. The accumulation of pro-inflammatory macrophages in tissues can lead to the development of various chronic inflammatory diseases, including rheumatoid arthritis, inflammatory bowel disease, and cardiovascular diseases, highlighting the need for targeted therapies that can modulate macrophage polarization and function [3].

2.3.3 Impact of inflammation-related diseases

The dysregulation of macrophage function during inflammation plays a significant role in the pathology of various diseases. For example, in cardiovascular diseases, activated macrophages infiltrate atherosclerotic plaques, contributing to plaque instability and the progression of atherosclerosis through the release of pro-inflammatory cytokines and matrix metalloproteinases [2]. Similarly, in cancer, tumor-associated macrophages (TAMs) can adopt an M2-like phenotype that supports tumor growth and metastasis by promoting angiogenesis and suppressing anti-tumor immune responses [12]. The presence of pro-inflammatory macrophages in chronic inflammatory diseases not only exacerbates tissue damage but also creates a microenvironment conducive to tumor development and progression [23]. Furthermore, the therapeutic targeting of macrophage polarization has emerged as a promising strategy for treating inflammation-related diseases. For instance, the modulation of macrophage activity through the use of small molecules, monoclonal antibodies, or gene therapy could potentially restore the balance between pro-inflammatory and anti-inflammatory macrophages, thereby alleviating disease symptoms and improving patient outcomes [3]. In conclusion, understanding the multifaceted roles of macrophages in inflammation is crucial for developing effective therapeutic strategies for a wide range of inflammatory diseases.

2.4 Macrophages and the tumor microenvironment

2.4.1 Characteristics of tumor-associated macrophages

Tumor-associated macrophages (TAMs) constitute a heterogeneous population of immune cells that are pivotal in the tumor microenvironment (TME). They exhibit remarkable plasticity, with functional states ranging from pro-inflammatory (M1) to anti-inflammatory (M2) phenotypes. The M1 phenotype is generally associated with anti-tumor immunity, characterized by the production of pro-inflammatory cytokines and antigen presentation capabilities, whereas the M2 phenotype is linked to tumor progression, promoting angiogenesis, tissue remodeling, and immunosuppression [24, 25]. This functional dichotomy is influenced by various factors within the TME, such as cytokines, growth factors, and metabolic signals. For example, hypoxic conditions within tumors can drive TAMs toward an M2-like phenotype, thereby aiding tumor growth and metastasis [26]. Furthermore, TAMs can be categorized based on their origin, with some originating from circulating monocytes and others from tissue-resident macrophages, which contributes to their functional diversity [27]. The interaction between TAMs and other components of the TME, such as cancer cells, fibroblasts, and the extracellular matrix, highlights their central role in shaping tumor biology and affecting therapeutic outcomes [28, 29].

2.4.2 Role of macrophages in tumor progression

Macrophages significantly influence tumor progression through various mechanisms, including modulation of immune responses, promotion of angiogenesis, and facilitation of metastasis. Within the TME, TAMs secrete a multitude of cytokines and growth factors that support tumor cell proliferation and create an immunosuppressive environment, hindering effective anti-tumor immune responses [25, 30]. For instance, TAMs produce vascular endothelial growth factor (VEGF) and other angiogenic factors that enhance blood vessel formation, supplying tumors with essential nutrients and oxygen. Additionally, TAMs can promote epithelial-to-mesenchymal transition (EMT) in cancer cells, a critical process for metastasis, by releasing transforming growth factor-beta (TGF-β) and other signaling molecules [28]. The presence of TAMs has been associated with poor prognosis in various cancers, including hepatocellular carcinoma and colorectal cancer, underscoring their role as key contributors to tumor aggressiveness and therapeutic resistance [29, 31]. Therefore, targeting TAMs to shift their function from pro-tumoral to anti-tumoral phenotypes represents a promising therapeutic approach in cancer treatment.

2.4.3 Targeting macrophages in immunotherapy

Considering the critical role of tumor-associated macrophages (TAMs) in tumor progression and immune evasion, they have become attractive targets for immunotherapy. Various strategies are being explored to modulate TAM function, including the use of small molecules, antibodies, and gene-editing technologies to reprogram macrophages toward an M1 phenotype [25, 30]. For example, therapies that inhibit the signaling pathways driving M2 polarization, such as the inhibition of IL-4 or IL-10, have shown promise in preclinical models [24]. Additionally, the use of checkpoint inhibitors has been investigated to enhance the anti-tumor activity of macrophages by reversing their immunosuppressive states [32]. Another innovative approach involves the use of nanoparticles or exosomes engineered to deliver therapeutic agents specifically to TAMs, thereby enhancing the efficacy of existing treatments [25, 28]. Clinical trials targeting TAMs are ongoing, and preliminary results indicate potential benefits when combined with traditional therapies, suggesting that a multifaceted approach to modulate the tumor microenvironment (TME) could improve patient outcomes in cancer therapy [31]. Overall, understanding the complex interactions between macrophages and the TME is essential for developing effective immunotherapeutic strategies against cancer.

2.5 The role of macrophages in autoimmune diseases

2.5.1 Pathological mechanisms of autoimmune diseases

Autoimmune diseases arise from a breakdown in immune tolerance mechanisms, leading to inappropriate immune responses to self-antigens. The core of these diseases' pathology is the dysregulation of immune cell functions, with macrophages playing a central role. As pivotal players in the immune system, macrophages can adopt various activation states that significantly influence their role in autoimmune pathology. In conditions such as rheumatoid arthritis and multiple sclerosis, macrophages are attracted to sites of inflammation where they can perpetuate tissue damage by releasing pro-inflammatory cytokines and mediators. The activation of macrophages is often triggered by the detection of self-antigens through pattern recognition receptors (PRRs), which can lead to the production of inflammatory mediators that exacerbate tissue injury and promote further immune cell recruitment [33, 34]. Additionally, the interaction between macrophages and other immune cells, such as T cells, can amplify the autoimmune response, creating a vicious cycle of inflammation and damage. This intricate interplay highlights the need for a deeper understanding of the cellular and molecular mechanisms that govern macrophage activation in autoimmune diseases, as it may uncover new therapeutic targets for restoring immune balance.

2.5.2 Dysfunction of macrophages

Macrophage dysfunction is a characteristic feature of autoimmune diseases, marked by altered polarization states and impaired efferocytosis. In autoimmune conditions, macrophages may become biased toward a pro-inflammatory phenotype (M1), which is associated with the production of inflammatory cytokines such as TNF-α and IL-6, further driving the inflammatory response [35, 36]. This shift in macrophage function not only contributes to local tissue damage but also disrupts systemic immune regulation, resulting in a failure to resolve inflammation. Moreover, defective efferocytosis—the process by which macrophages clear apoptotic cells—can exacerbate inflammation and autoimmunity. When apoptotic cells are not efficiently cleared, they can release autoantigens that further stimulate the immune response, perpetuating the cycle of inflammation and tissue damage [34, 37]. Understanding macrophage polarization and its implications in autoimmune diseases is crucial, as targeting these pathways may offer therapeutic avenues to restore macrophage function and mitigate disease progression.

2.5.3 Research progress in therapeutic interventions

Recent advances in therapeutic targeting of macrophages in autoimmune diseases have shown promising potential. Strategies aimed at modulating macrophage polarization, enhancing efferocytosis, and inhibiting pro-inflammatory pathways are being investigated. For example, the use of biologics targeting specific cytokines produced by activated macrophages, such as TNF-α inhibitors, has shown efficacy in conditions like rheumatoid arthritis [34, 38]. Additionally, emerging research on the role of long noncoding RNAs (lncRNAs) in regulating macrophage function suggests that these molecules could serve as novel therapeutic targets to modulate macrophage responses in autoimmune diseases [39]. Furthermore, the exploration of extracellular vesicles derived from macrophages as potential therapeutic agents is gaining

DOI: http://dx.doi.org/10.5772/intechopen.1012655

momentum, as these vesicles can carry anti-inflammatory signals and promote tissue repair [40]. Overall, ongoing research into the multifaceted roles of macrophages in autoimmune diseases underscores the importance of developing targeted therapies that can effectively restore immune homeostasis and alleviate disease symptoms.

2.6 Macrophage signaling pathways

2.6.1 The role of cytokines and receptors

Cytokines and their receptors are crucial in the signaling pathways that control macrophage function and polarization. Macrophages possess a range of receptors that enable them to respond to cytokines, which are essential for initiating and modulating immune responses. For example, the interaction of cytokines like Interleukin-6 (IL-6) with its receptor can result in various outcomes, depending on the activated signaling pathways. IL-6 can trigger classic signaling *via* membrane-bound receptors and trans-signaling through soluble receptors, leading to either pro-inflammatory or anti-inflammatory responses [41]. The complexity of these interactions is further emphasized by the presence of various pattern recognition receptors (PRRs), macrophages are able to detect pathogens and tissue damage. These receptors, which include Toll-like receptors (TLRs), activate intracellular pathways such as NF-κB and MAPK, which are vital for the production of pro-inflammatory cytokines and chemokines [42]. Additionally, the balance between pro-inflammatory (M1) and anti-inflammatory (M2) macrophage polarization is significantly affected by the cytokine environment. For example, TNF-α and IL-1β are pivotal in promoting M1 polarization, whereas IL-4 and IL-10 support M2 polarization, underscoring the critical role of cytokines in shaping macrophage destiny and function in both health and disease [25, 43]. Comprehending these signaling dynamics is fundamental for the development of targeted therapies aimed at adjusting macrophage activity in various diseases, including autoimmune conditions and cancer.

2.6.2 Regulation of signaling pathways

The regulation of macrophage signaling pathways is a complex and dynamic process that involves various intracellular mechanisms. Key signaling pathways, such as the NF-κB, JAK/STAT, and MAPK pathways, are crucial for mediating macrophage responses to cytokines and other stimuli. For instance, the NF-κB pathway is activated upon engagement of PRRs by pathogens or cytokines, leading to the transcription of pro-inflammatory genes [43]. This pathway's regulation is tightly controlled by various feedback mechanisms, including the action of negative regulators such as IκB proteins, which sequester NF-κB in the cytoplasm. Additionally, the JAK/STAT pathway, particularly STAT3, plays a significant role in mediating the effects of IL-6 and IL-10, promoting anti-inflammatory responses and M2 polarization [41]. Furthermore, metabolic reprogramming within macrophages is increasingly recognized as a regulatory mechanism that influences signaling pathways. For example, the metabolic shift from oxidative phosphorylation to glycolysis in M1 macrophages enhances their inflammatory capabilities, while M2 macrophages exhibit increased oxidative metabolism, supporting tissue repair and resolution of inflammation [42]. This interplay between metabolic state and signaling pathways highlights potential therapeutic targets for modulating macrophage function in various diseases, including chronic inflammatory conditions and cancer.

2.6.3 Metabolic reprogramming and functional regulation

Metabolic reprogramming is a critical aspect of macrophage activation and function, influencing their roles in both homeostasis and disease. When macrophages encounter pathogens or inflammatory signals, they undergo metabolic shifts that enable them to meet the energy demands of their activated state. M1 macrophages typically exhibit increased glycolysis and lactate production, which supports rapid proliferation and the synthesis of pro-inflammatory mediators [42, 43]. In contrast, M2 macrophages favor oxidative phosphorylation and fatty acid oxidation, reflecting their role in tissue repair and anti-inflammatory responses. This metabolic plasticity is regulated by various signaling pathways, including AMPK and mTOR, which sense changes in nutrient availability and energy status [42]. Moreover, recent studies have identified specific metabolites, such as succinate and itaconate, that can modulate macrophage signaling and function, further emphasizing the importance of metabolic pathways in shaping immune responses [42]. The understanding of how metabolic reprogramming influences macrophage polarization and function opens new avenues for therapeutic interventions aimed at modulating macrophage activity in diseases characterized by chronic inflammation, such as obesity, diabetes, and cancer. By targeting metabolic pathways, it may be possible to enhance the resolution of inflammation or promote the anti-tumor activities of macrophages, thereby improving clinical outcomes in various pathological conditions.

2.7 Macrophage cross-species research

2.7.1 Research progress in mouse models

Mouse models have been pivotal in advancing our understanding of macrophage biology, particularly in the context of both physiological and pathological processes. These models allow researchers to manipulate genetic and environmental variables to observe changes in macrophage behavior and function. For instance, studies utilizing genetically modified mice have elucidated the roles of specific genes in macrophage activation and polarization. One notable advancement is the use of transgenic mouse models that express fluorescent markers in macrophages, enabling real-time visualization of these cells during inflammatory responses. This has facilitated the investigation of macrophage dynamics in various disease models, such as atherosclerosis and cancer. The application of advanced imaging techniques, including intravital microscopy, has provided insights into the interactions between macrophages and other cell types within live tissues. For instance, researchers have shown that macrophages can directly affect the behavior of tumor cells, promoting either tumor progression or regression depending on their polarization state. Additionally, the use of mouse models has enabled the testing of novel therapeutic approaches targeting macrophages, such as modulating their polarization through pharmacological agents or genetic interventions. Overall, mouse models remain an invaluable tool for unraveling the complex biology of macrophages and their roles in health and disease [44, 45].

2.7.2 Characteristics of human macrophages

Human macrophages exhibit a significant degree of heterogeneity, influenced by their tissue microenvironment and the specific signals they encounter. Unlike mouse macrophages, which are often studied in isolation, human macrophages exist within a complex network of interactions with other immune and non-immune cells. This complexity is particularly evident in tissues such as the lungs and liver, where macrophages play critical roles in maintaining homeostasis and responding to injury. Human macrophages can be broadly categorized into pro-inflammatory M1 and anti-inflammatory M2 phenotypes, each characterized by distinct functional capabilities and metabolic profiles. Recent studies have emphasized the importance of macrophage plasticity, demonstrating that these cells can rapidly switch between phenotypes in response to changing environmental cues. For example, in the context of chronic diseases such as obesity and diabetes, macrophages in adipose tissue can adopt a pro-inflammatory state that contributes to insulin resistance. Conversely, during tissue repair, macrophages may shift toward an M2 phenotype to promote healing and resolution of inflammation. Furthermore, the study of human macrophages has uncovered unique surface markers and secretory profiles that distinguish them from their murine counterparts, underscoring the necessity of using human models to accurately reflect macrophage behavior in clinical settings. This understanding is crucial for developing targeted therapies aimed at modulating macrophage function in various diseases [46, 47].

2.7.3 Significance of comparative studies

Comparative studies between human and mouse macrophages are essential for translating preclinical findings into clinical applications. These studies not only highlight the similarities and differences in macrophage biology across species but also inform the development of more effective therapeutic strategies. For example, while mouse models have provided significant insights into the mechanisms of macrophage activation and polarization, discrepancies in macrophage responses between species can complicate the prediction of human outcomes. This is particularly relevant in the context of drug development, where therapies that are effective in mouse models may not produce the same results in human patients. Comparative research has also revealed that certain signaling pathways and regulatory mechanisms may be conserved across species, while others may be uniquely adapted to human physiology. Understanding these nuances is crucial for identifying potential therapeutic targets that can be effectively manipulated in humans. Moreover, the integration of advanced technologies such as single-cell RNA sequencing and mass spectrometry in comparative studies has enhanced our ability to dissect the functional diversity of macrophages at an unprecedented resolution. This knowledge not only advances our understanding of macrophage biology but also paves the way for innovative approaches to treat diseases characterized by macrophage dysfunction, such as cancer and autoimmune disorders [48, 49].

2.8 The therapeutic potential of macrophages

2.8.1 Macrophages as drug targets

Macrophages have emerged as significant therapeutic targets due to their pivotal role in various physiological and pathological processes. Their ability to adopt distinct functional phenotypes, primarily categorized as M1 (pro-inflammatory) and M2 (anti-inflammatory), makes them crucial in mediating immune responses and tissue homeostasis. This phenotypic plasticity is influenced by the microenvironment, which can be manipulated to enhance therapeutic outcomes. For instance, targeting specific signaling pathways that regulate macrophage polarization can shift the balance toward the M2 phenotype, promoting tissue repair and reducing inflammation in diseases such as rheumatoid arthritis and atherosclerosis [50, 51]. Additionally, the development of novel drug delivery systems that specifically target macrophages enhances the efficacy of therapeutic agents while minimizing systemic side effects. For example, liposomal formulations modified with ligands that bind to macrophage surface receptors have shown promise in delivering anti-inflammatory drugs directly to inflamed tissues, thereby improving treatment outcomes in conditions like ulcerative colitis and chronic inflammatory diseases [51, 52]. Furthermore, the identification of macrophage-specific markers and the use of nanotechnology to create targeted therapies represent exciting avenues for enhancing the specificity and effectiveness of treatments aimed at modulating macrophage function in various diseases.

2.8.2 Prospects for cell therapy applications

The application of macrophages in cell therapy presents a novel approach to treating a range of diseases, particularly those characterized by chronic inflammation or immune dysregulation. Recent advances in regenerative medicine have highlighted the potential of using engineered macrophages to restore tissue homeostasis and promote healing. For instance, the reprogramming of macrophages to adopt an anti-inflammatory phenotype has been explored as a therapeutic strategy in conditions such as myocardial infarction and neurodegenerative diseases [15, 53]. Moreover, the use of induced pluripotent stem cell-derived macrophages (iMacs) offers a promising platform for personalized medicine, allowing for the generation of patient-specific macrophages that can be tailored to target specific disease mechanisms [54]. These iMacs can be utilized to study disease pathogenesis, screen for drugs, and develop novel therapeutic strategies that leverage the unique properties of macrophages. Additionally, combining macrophage-based therapies with other modalities, such as gene editing or immunotherapy, may enhance their therapeutic efficacy and broaden their application across various conditions, including cancer and autoimmune diseases [27, 55].

2.8.3 Future research directions

Future research on macrophages should concentrate on clarifying the complex mechanisms behind their functional plasticity and the interplay between their metabolic states and phenotypes. Understanding how metabolic pathways affect macrophage polarization and function will be crucial for developing targeted therapies that can modulate macrophage activity in disease contexts. Moreover, exploring the heterogeneity of macrophages within various tissue microenvironments and their responses to different stimuli will offer insights into their roles in health and disease [17, 20]. Additionally, the incorporation of advanced technologies such as single-cell transcriptomics and metabolomics will enable a more comprehensive understanding of macrophage biology and their interactions with other immune cells and the extracellular matrix. This knowledge can propel the development of innovative therapeutic strategies that leverage the unique properties of macrophages, ultimately leading to enhanced treatment outcomes for a broad spectrum of inflammatory and degenerative diseases. Lastly, clinical trials assessing macrophage-targeted therapies will be vital to ensure their safety and efficacy in human populations, facilitating their adoption into standard clinical practice.

2.9 Advances in macrophage research

2.9.1 Single-cell sequencing technology

Single-cell sequencing technology has revolutionized our understanding of macrophage biology by enabling the detailed analysis of individual cells within heterogeneous populations. This approach allows researchers to dissect the complex phenotypic and functional diversity of macrophages, which are crucial for immune responses and tissue homeostasis. This approach has recently utilized single-cell RNA sequencing (scRNA-seq) to identify distinct macrophage subpopulations and their specific roles in various physiological and pathological contexts, such as inflammation, cancer, and tissue repair [56, 57]. For instance, the application of scRNA-seq has revealed unique transcriptional profiles associated with macrophage polarization, highlighting the dynamic nature of these cells in response to microenvironmental cues [3]. Moreover, this technology has facilitated the identification of novel macrophage-associated biomarkers and therapeutic targets, paving the way for more personalized approaches in treating diseases linked to macrophage dysfunction [10]. By integrating single-cell transcriptomics with other omics technologies, researchers can gain a comprehensive understanding of macrophage metabolism, signaling pathways, and interactions with other immune cells, thus advancing our knowledge of their roles in health and disease [58].

2.9.2 Application of imaging technologies

Imaging technologies have become indispensable tools in macrophage research, allowing for real-time visualization of these cells *in vivo* and providing insights into their dynamic behaviors and interactions within tissues. Techniques such as positron emission tomography (PET) and two-photon microscopy have enabled researchers to track macrophage migration, activation, and polarization in various pathological conditions, including cardiovascular diseases and cancer [21, 22]. For example, PET imaging has been successfully used to quantify macrophage accumulation in inflamed tissues, offering a non-invasive method to assess disease progression and response to therapies [15]. Additionally, advanced imaging modalities facilitate the study of macrophage interactions with other cell types, such as endothelial cells and fibroblasts, within the tumor microenvironment, thereby elucidating the complex cellular networks that drive inflammation and tissue remodeling [3, 59]. The integration of imaging technologies with molecular probes that specifically target macrophage markers further enhances the ability to monitor their functional states and assess therapeutic efficacy in real-time, ultimately contributing to the development of macrophage-targeted therapies [15].

2.9.3 Construction and application of in vitro models

The construction of *in vitro* models has significantly advanced our understanding of macrophage biology by providing controlled environments to study their differentiation, activation, and interactions with other cell types. Recent innovations include the development of three-dimensional (3D) culture systems that better mimic the physiological conditions of tissues, allowing for more accurate assessments of macrophage function and behavior [60]. For example, 3D organoid models have been utilized to study macrophage responses to various stimuli, including pathogens and inflammatory signals, revealing insights into their role in tissue homeostasis and disease [61]. Additionally, co-culture systems that incorporate macrophages with other cell types, such as fibroblasts or endothelial cells, have proven valuable for investigating the complex cellular interactions that occur during inflammation and tissue repair [62]. These *in vitro* models not only facilitate the exploration of macrophage polarization and functional plasticity but also serve as platforms for testing potential therapeutic agents aimed at modulating macrophage activity in various diseases [56]. By leveraging these advanced models, researchers can gain deeper insights into the mechanisms underlying macrophage-mediated pathologies and identify novel therapeutic strategies to target these critical immune cells effectively.

3. Conclusion

Macrophages play a crucial role in both physiological and pathological processes, exhibiting remarkable versatility in their functions. As we have discussed throughout this chapter, the complex characteristics and mechanisms of action of macrophages have significant implications for our understanding of various diseases, ranging from chronic inflammatory conditions to cancer. The dual roles of macrophages—as facilitators of tissue homeostasis and contributors to disease pathology—necessitate a nuanced appreciation of their behavior in different contexts.

The research landscape surrounding macrophages has evolved significantly, driven by advances in technology and a deeper understanding of cellular biology. The identification of distinct macrophage phenotypes and their functional plasticity has opened new avenues for therapeutic intervention. For example, the recognition of pro-inflammatory M1 macrophages versus anti-inflammatory M2 macrophages has underscored the importance of macrophage polarization in determining disease outcomes. This polarization is not static; rather, it reflects a dynamic response to local microenvironments and systemic signals. Future studies should focus on elucidating the triggers and pathways that govern these transitions, as this knowledge could inform strategies for modulating macrophage activity in disease contexts.

Moreover, the influence of macrophages extends beyond their direct interactions with other immune cells. Their function within the tumor microenvironment highlights the complexity of macrophage biology, as they can either foster tumor growth and metastasis or provoke anti-tumor responses. This duality poses a challenge for therapeutic strategies aimed at utilizing macrophages for cancer treatment. Achieving a balance between promoting beneficial macrophage activities and reducing their potential to worsen the disease necessitates a thorough comprehension of the signaling pathways that govern macrophage activation and differentiation.

As researchers persist in exploring the diverse roles of macrophages, it is crucial to integrate findings from various disciplines, including immunology, oncology, and regenerative medicine. Cross-disciplinary collaboration will enhance our understanding of macrophage biology and facilitate the translation of basic research into clinical applications. For instance, the exploration of macrophage-targeted therapies, such as the use of nanoparticles for drug delivery, highlights the potential for innovative treatment strategies that can improve patient outcomes across a range of diseases.

Moreover, the development of personalized medicine approaches necessitates consideration of individual variability in macrophage function. Genetic, epigenetic, and environmental factors can influence macrophage behavior, and understanding these variations will be essential for tailoring therapies to individual patients.

Moving forward, it will be important to establish robust biomarkers that can predict macrophage responses in various disease states, allowing for more precise therapeutic interventions.

In conclusion, the multifaceted roles of macrophages in health and disease represent a promising frontier in biomedical research. Continued investigation into the dynamic changes of macrophages in various pathological conditions will not only enhance our understanding of disease mechanisms but also pave the way for novel therapeutic strategies. By fostering a holistic view that balances different research perspectives and findings, we can unlock the full potential of macrophage-targeted therapies, ultimately contributing to more effective prevention and treatment options for a variety of diseases. The ongoing evolution of macrophage research holds great promise, and the insights gained will undoubtedly shape the future of clinical practice in profound and meaningful ways.

Author details

Yan Chen* and Teng Li
Urology Department, The First Affiliated Hospital of Zhengzhou University, Zhengzhou, China

*Address all correspondence to: chenyan.abby@163.com

References

[1] Jiang S, Yang H, Li M. Emerging roles of lysophosphatidic acid in macrophages and inflammatory diseases. International Journal of Molecular Sciences. 2023;**24**(15):12524. DOI: 10.3390/ijms241512524

[2] Chen J, Zhu Z, Wang Y, Yu J, Zhang X, Xu Y. Cardiac resident macrophages in cardiovascular disease: From physiology to pathology. Heart. 2025;**111**(9):391-400. DOI: 10.1136/heartjnl-2024-324333

[3] Clevenger AJ, Jha A, Moore E, Raghavan SA. Manipulating immune activity of macrophages: A materials and mechanics perspective. Trends in Biotechnology. 2025;**43**(1):131-144. DOI: 10.1016/j.tibtech.2024.07.009

[4] Orliaguet L, Ejlalmanesh T, Alzaid F. Metabolic and molecular mechanisms of macrophage polarisation and adipose tissue insulin resistance. International Journal of Molecular Sciences. 2020;**21**(16):5731. DOI: 10.3390/ijms21165731

[5] Sekine H, Takeda H, Takeda N, et al. PNPO-PLP axis senses prolonged hypoxia in macrophages by regulating lysosomal activity. Nature Metabolism. 2024;**6**(6):1108-1127. DOI: 10.1038/s42255-024-01053-4

[6] Zhang XM, Chen DG, Li SC, Zhu B, Li ZJ. Embryonic origin and subclonal evolution of tumor-associated macrophages imply preventive care for cancer. Cells. 2021;**10**(4):903. DOI: 10.3390/cells10040903

[7] Moadab F, Khorramdelazad H, Abbasifard M. Role of CCL2/CCR2 axis in the immunopathogenesis of rheumatoid arthritis: Latest evidence and therapeutic approaches. Life Sciences. 2021;**269**:119034. DOI: 10.1016/j.lfs.2021.119034

[8] Son CJ, Carnino JM, Lee H, Jin Y. Emerging roles of circular RNA in macrophage activation and inflammatory lung responses. Cells. 2024;**13**(17):1407. DOI: 10.3390/cells13171407

[9] Lv H, Sun H, Wang L, et al. Targeting CD301^{+} macrophages inhibits endometrial fibrosis and improves pregnancy outcome. EMBO Molecular Medicine. 2023;**15**(9):e17601. DOI: 10.15252/emmm.202317601

[10] Khayati S, Dehnavi S, Sadeghi M, Tavakol Afshari J, Esmaeili SA, Mohammadi M. The potential role of miRNA in regulating macrophage polarization. Heliyon. 2023;**9**(11):e21615. DOI: 10.1016/j.heliyon.2023.e21615

[11] Akkız H. Emerging role of cancer-associated fibroblasts in progression and treatment of hepatocellular carcinoma. International Journal of Molecular Sciences. 2023;**24**(4):3941. DOI: 10.3390/ijms24043941

[12] Marelli G, Morina N, Portale F, et al. Lipid-loaded macrophages as new therapeutic target in cancer. Journal for Immunotherapy of Cancer. 2022;**10**(7):e004584. DOI: 10.1136/jitc-2022-004584

[13] Abuawad A, Mbadugha C, Ghaemmaghami AM, Kim DH. Metabolic characterisation of THP-1 macrophage polarisation using LC-MS-based metabolite profiling. Metabolomics. 2020;**16**(3):33. DOI: 10.1007/s11306-020-01656-4

[14] Lu YZ, Nayer B, Singh SK, Alshoubaki YK, Yuan E, Park AJ,

et al. CGRP sensory neurons promote tissue healing via neutrophils and macrophages. Nature. 2024;**628**(8008):604-611. DOI: 10.1038/s41586-024-07237-y

[15] Yoshino O, Ono Y. The physiological role of macrophages in reproductive organs. Reproductive Medicine and Biology. 2025;**24**(1):e12637. DOI: 10.1002/rmb2.12637

[16] Consonni FM, Incerti M, Bertolotti M, Ballerini G, Garlatti V, Sica A. Heme catabolism and heme oxygenase-1-expressing myeloid cells in pathophysiology. Frontiers in Immunology. 2024;**15**:1433113. DOI: 10.3389/fimmu.2024.1433113

[17] Cheng J, Cai W, Zong S, Yu Y, Wei F. Metabolite transporters as regulators of macrophage polarization. Naunyn-Schmiedeberg's Archives of Pharmacology. 2022;**395**(1):13-25. DOI: 10.1007/s00210-021-02173-4

[18] Lee E, Eo JC, Lee C, Yu JW. Distinct features of brain-resident macrophages: Microglia and non-parenchymal brain macrophages. Molecules and Cells. 2021;**44**(5):281-291. DOI: 10.14348/molcells.2021.0060. Available from: https://pubmed.ncbi.nlm.nih.gov/33972475/

[19] Sheng YR, Hu WT, Chen S, Zhu XY. Efferocytosis by macrophages in physiological and pathological conditions: Regulatory pathways and molecular mechanisms. Frontiers in Immunology. 2024;**15**:1275203. DOI: 10.3389/fimmu.2024.1275203

[20] Li S, Wu YR, Peng XQ, et al. A novel cargo delivery system-AnCar-Exo^{LaIMTS} ameliorates arthritis via specifically targeting pro-inflammatory macrophages. Advanced Science (Weinh). 2024;**11**(7):e2306143. DOI: 10.1002/advs.202306143

[21] Hao W, Chen S, Chao H, et al. IL-33-induced TREM2^{+} macrophages promote pathological new bone formation through CREG1-IGF2R axis in ankylosing spondylitis. Advanced Science (Weinh). 2025;**12**(18):e2500952. DOI: 10.1002/advs.202500952

[22] Atsumi Y, Toriyama M, Kato H, et al. Anti-inflammatory role of TRPV4 in human macrophages. Immunohorizons. 2023;7(1):81-96. DOI: 10.4049/immunohorizons.2200100

[23] Geyer CE, Mes L, Newling M, den Dunnen J, Hoepel W. Physiological and pathological inflammation induced by antibodies and pentraxins. Cells. 2021;**10**(5):1175. DOI: 10.3390/cells10051175

[24] Lu L, Liu YJ, Cheng PQ, Hu D, Xu HC, Ji G. Macrophages play a role in inflammatory transformation of colorectal cancer. World Journal of Gastrointestinal Oncology. 2021;**13**(12):2013-2028. DOI: 10.4251/wjgo.v13.i12.2013

[25] Li SY, Guo YL, Tian JW, et al. Anti-tumor strategies by harnessing the phagocytosis of macrophages. Cancers (Basel). 2023;**15**(10):2717. DOI: 10.3390/cancers15102717

[26] Dong Y, Yang Q, Niu R, et al. Modulation of tumor-associated macrophages in colitis-associated colorectal cancer. Journal of Cellular Physiology. 2022;**237**(12):4443-4459. DOI: 10.1002/jcp.30906

[27] Karimova AF, Ketkar A, Suezov R, et al. In vitro functional assays to assess the reciprocal interplay between tumor cells and macrophages. The FASEB Journal. 2024;**38**(13):e23730. DOI: 10.1096/fj.202400240R

[28] Zhou Z, Wang Z, Gao J, et al. Noncoding RNA-mediated macrophage and cancer cell crosstalk in hepatocellular carcinoma. Molecular Therapy - Oncolytics. 2022;**25**:98-120. DOI: 10.1016/j.omto.2022.03.002

[29] Guan Y, Zhang M, Song J, et al. CaMKK2 regulates macrophage polarization induced by matrix stiffness: Implications for shaping the immune response in stiffened tissues. Advanced Science (Weinh). 2025;**12**(16):e2417778. DOI: 10.1002/advs.202417778

[30] Zhang L, Chen C, Feng J, Zhang H, Nguyen LXT, Chen Z. The role of YTHDF2 in anti-tumor immunity. Cell Investigation. 2025;**1**(1):100008. DOI: 10.1016/j.clnves.2025.100008

[31] Gryziak M, Kraj L, Stec R. The role of tumor-associated macrophages in hepatocellular carcinoma-from bench to bedside: A review. Journal of Gastroenterology and Hepatology. 2024;**39**(8):1489-1499. DOI: 10.1111/jgh.16564

[32] Liu H, Pan M, Liu M, et al. Lactate: A rising star in tumors and inflammation. Frontiers in Immunology. 2024;**15**:1496390. DOI: 10.3389/fimmu.2024.1496390

[33] Liang HY, Chen Y, Wei X, et al. Immunomodulatory functions of TRPM7 and its implications in autoimmune diseases. Immunology. 2022;**165**(1):3-21. DOI: 10.1111/imm.13420

[34] Yang Y, Han X, Sun L, Shao F, Yin Y, Zhang W. ETS transcription factors in immune cells and immune-related diseases. International Journal of Molecular Sciences. 2024;**25**(18):10004. DOI: 10.3390/ijms251810004

[35] Singh A, Behl T, Sehgal A, et al. Exploring the therapeutic promise of targeting rho kinase in rheumatoid arthritis. Inflammopharmacology. 2021;**29**(6):1641-1651. DOI: 10.1007/s10787-021-00884-x

[36] Yang H, Luo Y, Lai X. The comprehensive role of apoptosis inhibitor of macrophage (AIM) in pathological conditions. Clinical and Experimental Immunology. 2023;**212**(3):184-198. DOI: 10.1093/cei/uxac095

[37] Razi S, Yaghmoorian Khojini J, Kargarijam F, et al. Macrophage efferocytosis in health and disease. Cell Biochemistry and Function. 2023;**41**(2):152-165. DOI: 10.1002/cbf.3780

[38] Li X, Li S, Fu X, Wang Y. Apoptotic extracellular vesicles restore homeostasis of the articular microenvironment for the treatment of rheumatoid arthritis. Bioactive Materials. 2024;**35**:564-576. DOI: 10.1016/j.bioactmat.2023.11.019

[39] Zhao Q, Pang G, Yang L, Chen S, Xu R, Shao W. Long noncoding RNAs regulate the inflammatory responses of macrophages. Cells. 2021;**11**(1):5. DOI: 10.3390/cells11010005

[40] Zhou M, Liu W, Zhang J, Sun N. RNA m^6A modification in immunocytes and DNA repair: The biological functions and prospects in clinical application. Frontiers in Cell and Development Biology. 2021;**9**:794754. DOI: 10.3389/fcell.2021.794754

[41] García-Juárez M, Camacho-Morales A. Defining the role of anti- and pro-inflammatory outcomes of interleukin-6 in mental health. Neuroscience. 2022;**492**:32-46. DOI: 10.1016/j.neuroscience.2022.03.020

[42] Escalona E, Olate-Briones A, Albornoz-Muñoz S, et al. Neu1 deficiency and fibrotic lymph

node microenvironment lead to imbalance in M1/M2 macrophage polarization. Frontiers in Immunology. 2024;**15**:1462853. DOI: 10.3389/fimmu.2024.1462853

[43] Sun Z, Ke P, Shen Y, et al. MXRA7 is involved in monocyte-to-macrophage differentiation. Molecular Immunology. 2024;**171**:12-21. DOI: 10.1016/j.molimm.2024.05.001

[44] Shrestha KR, Kim S, Jo A, Ragothaman M, Yoo SY. *In vivo* safety evaluation and tracing of arginylglycylaspartic acid-engineered phage nanofiber in murine model. Journal of Materials Chemistry B. 2024;**12**(40):10258-10271. DOI: 10.1039/d4tb00823e

[45] Gurney M, Davies LC, Jones RE, et al. Lentiviral vector preparation for efficient gene and microRNA modulation of peritoneal cavity tissue-resident macrophages in vivo in mice. Journal of Visualized Experiments. 16 Feb 2024;(204). DOI: 10.3791/64926

[46] Sheng W, Ji G, Zhang L. Role of macrophage scavenger receptor MSR1 in the progression of non-alcoholic steatohepatitis. Frontiers in Immunology. 2022;**13**:1050984. DOI: 10.3389/fimmu.2022.1050984

[47] Lu C, Liao S, Chen B, et al. Responsive probes for in vivo magnetic resonance imaging of nitric oxide. Nature Materials. 2025;**24**(1):133-142. DOI: 10.1038/s41563-024-02054-0

[48] Amalia SN, Baral H, Fujiwara C, et al. TRPV4 regulates the development of psoriasis by controlling adenosine triphosphate expression in keratinocytes and the neuroimmune system. The Journal of Investigative Dermatology. 2023;**143**(12):2356-2365.e5. DOI: 10.1016/j.jid.2023.05.009

[49] He D, Li X, Zhang F, et al. Dec2 inhibits macrophage pyroptosis to promote periodontal homeostasis. Journal of Periodontal and Implant Science. 2022;**52**(1):28-38. DOI: 10.5051/jpis.2101380069

[50] Zhou X, Huang D, Wang R, et al. Targeted therapy of rheumatoid arthritis via macrophage repolarization. Drug Delivery. 2021;**28**(1):2447-2459. DOI: 10.1080/10717544.2021.2000679

[51] Liu M, Yao C, Liu S, et al. Intelligent response micelles with high andrographolide loading for the effective treatment of atherosclerosis. International Journal of Pharmaceutics. 2024;**665**:124705. DOI: 10.1016/j.ijpharm.2024.124705

[52] Zhang Y, Ma R, You C, et al. Hyaluronic acid modified oral drug delivery system with mucoadhesiveness and macrophage-targeting for colitis treatment. Carbohydrate Polymers. 2023;**313**:120884. DOI: 10.1016/j.carbpol.2023.120884

[53] Xu D, Bi S, Li J, et al. Legumain-guided Ferulate-peptide self-assembly enhances macrophage-endotheliocyte partnership to promote therapeutic angiogenesis after myocardial infarction. Advanced Healthcare Materials. 2024;**13**(30):e2402056. DOI: 10.1002/adhm.202402056

[54] Tiwari SK, Wong WJ, Moreira M, Pasqualini C, Ginhoux F. Induced pluripotent stem cell-derived macrophages as a platform for modelling human disease. Nature Reviews. Immunology. 2025;**25**(2):108-124. DOI: 10.1038/s41577-024-01081-x

[55] Chen X, Li P, Wang G. Development of a fluorescent probe for detecting superoxide anions for monitoring the progression and treatment of acute

spondylitis. Analytical Methods. 2025;**17**(3):533-538. DOI: 10.1039/d4ay01626b

[56] Hu X, Liu X, Feng D, et al. Polarization of macrophages in tumor microenvironment using high-throughput single-cell metabolomics. Analytical Chemistry. 2024;**96**(37):14935-14943. DOI: 10.1021/acs.analchem.4c02989

[57] Gallo PM, Elliott E, Ford GC, et al. The protective role of transcription factor Nrf2 in murine macrophage activation syndrome. Journal of Leukocyte Biology. 2025;**117**(3):qiae225. DOI: 10.1093/jleuko/qiae225

[58] Del Barrio CC, Bindila L. Integrated cellular 4D-TIMS lipidomics and transcriptomics for characterization of anti-inflammatory and anti-atherosclerotic phenotype of MyD88-KO macrophages. Frontiers in Cell and Development Biology. 2024;**12**:1450971. DOI: 10.3389/fcell.2024.1450971

[59] Li G, Wu M, Chen K, et al. ROS-mediated M1 polarization-necroptosis crosstalk involved in Di-(2-ethylhexyl) phthalate-induced chicken liver injury. Poultry Science. 2025;**104**(1):104558. DOI: 10.1016/j.psj.2024.104558

[60] Arlat A, Renoud ML, Nakhle J, et al. Generation of functionally active resident macrophages from adipose tissue by 3D cultures. Frontiers in Immunology. 2024;**15**:1356397. DOI: 10.3389/fimmu.2024.1356397

[61] Ren X, He J, Hu H, Kohsaka S, Zhao LR. Hematopoietic growth factors regulate entry of monocytes into the adult brain via chemokine receptor CCR5. bioRxiv [Preprint]. 15 May 2024:2024.05.15.594359. DOI: 10.1101/2024.05.15.594359

[62] Li X, Zhu L. Comprehensive profiling of cell type-specific expression and distribution of complement genes in mouse and human kidneys: Insights into normal physiology and response to kidney transplantations. Renal Failure. 2025;**47**(1):2471568. DOI: 10.1080/0886022X.2025.2471568

Section 3

Macrophages in Infectious Diseases

Chapter 3

Phagocytes as Key Players: Unveiling Cell-Death Patterns Induced by Vaccines in Combating Infectious Diseases

Paulo R.Z. Antas

Abstract

This chapter delves into an in-depth analysis of the central role played by phagocytes—particularly macrophages—in modulating immune responses elicited by vaccines against infectious diseases. It emphasizes the functional plasticity and immunological versatility of macrophages, focusing on their capacity to integrate signals from vaccine-induced cell-death pathways, including apoptosis, necrosis, and pyroptosis. These cell-death modalities are examined in the context of their capacity to influence antigen availability, inflammatory milieu, and subsequent immune activation. Here, macrophages are further characterized beyond their canonical role in pathogen clearance, with detailed attention to their contributions to antigen processing and presentation, cytokine and chemokine secretion, tissue remodeling, and the orchestration of both innate and adaptive immune responses. Particular emphasis is placed on their immunoregulatory functions in viral pathogenesis and vaccine responsiveness. The chapter also interrogates the bidirectional crosstalk between vaccine-induced cell death and macrophage activation states, delineating how this interplay shapes immunogenicity and vaccine efficacy. It explores the translational implications of these findings for rational vaccine design, including strategies to potentiate macrophage-mediated immunomodulation through targeted adjuvants or delivery systems. By elucidating the mechanistic underpinnings of macrophage involvement in vaccine-induced immunity, this chapter aims to inform the development of next-generation vaccines that leverage programmed cell-death pathways to optimize immunological outcomes and therapeutic efficacy.

Keywords: phagocytes, cell-death, vaccines, infectious diseases, immune response

1. Introduction

The mononuclear phagocyte system (MPS), comprising monocytes and macrophages, constitutes a fundamental component of the host immune defense. Nonetheless, macrophages are particularly indispensable to the immunological response elicited by vaccination. These cells play a central role in orchestrating immune responses to diverse vaccine platforms, thereby contributing to protective immunity against a broad spectrum of infectious agents. As professional phagocytes, MPS constituents are not only first-line responders to invading pathogens but also serve as critical regulators of immune homeostasis, inflammation, and tissue regeneration. In the context of vaccination, macrophages are instrumental in antigen processing and presentation, cytokine secretion, and the execution of various forms of programmed cell death (PCD), all of which collectively shape the immunological milieu. The relevance of these functions is underscored by their involvement in the efficacy of several licensed vaccines targeting pathogens where MPS cells are key immunological mediators. This chapter centers on these immunobiological dynamics.

Beyond antigen presentation, MPS cells are actively engaged in immunomodulatory cell-death pathways that potentiate vaccine-induced immune responses (**Figure 1**). These cells can undergo multiple forms of PCD—including apoptosis, autophagy, netosis, pyroptosis, necroptosis, and ferroptosis—each contributing uniquely to pathogen control and immune regulation [1, 2]. Apoptosis, a non-inflammatory form of PCD, facilitates the clearance of infected or damaged cells while preserving tissue integrity and promoting immune tolerance [1]. Autophagy, a catabolic process involving the lysosomal degradation of cytoplasmic components, plays a dual role in innate and adaptive immunity by eliminating intracellular pathogens and enhancing antigen presentation [2]. Netosis, predominantly observed in neutrophils, entails the release of neutrophil extracellular traps (NETs) composed of chromatin

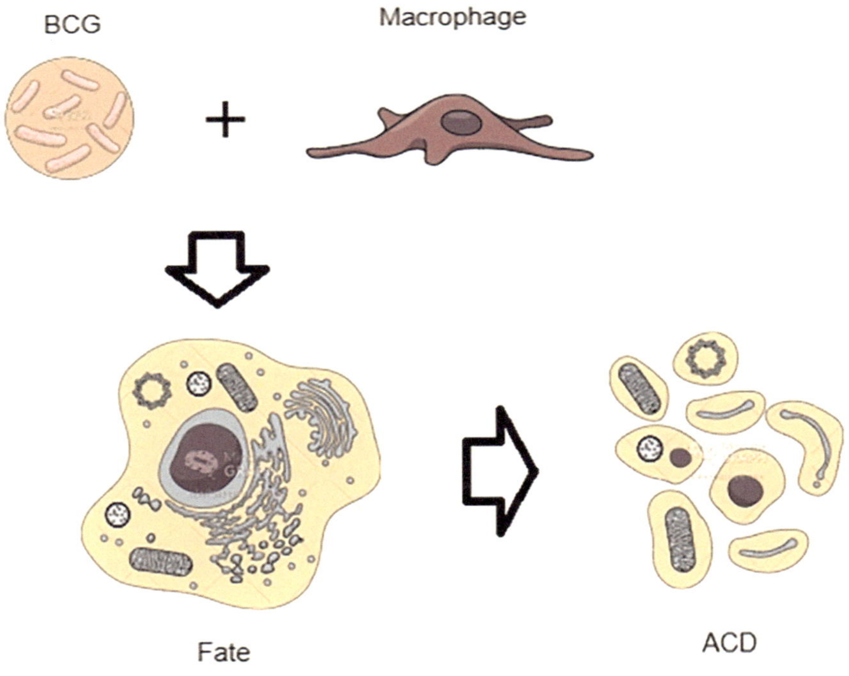

Figure 1.
Sequence of interactions and transformations involving a prototype vaccine (e.g., Bacillus Calmette-Guérin or BCG) and a mononuclear phagocyte system member (e.g., MPS = macrophage), leading to a programmed cell death (PCD). 1. BCG vaccine vs. MPS interaction: BCG (left) interacts with a macrophage (right); 2. Engulfment: The macrophage engulfs BCG, initiating the cellular fate process; 3. PCD: The final stage shows scattered, multiple apoptotic bodies after specific cell death. Generated by the Mind the Graph app.

and antimicrobial proteins, which immobilize and neutralize pathogens [3]. Pyroptosis, in contrast, is a lytic and pro-inflammatory form of cell death that amplifies immune signaling and pathogen clearance [1]. Necroptosis and ferroptosis also contribute to the elimination of infected cells and the modulation of inflammatory responses [1, 2].

In addition to their roles in cell death, MPS cells are integral to broader immunological processes. They modulate immune responses through cytokine production and crosstalk with other immune cell subsets, thereby coordinating and amplifying host defense mechanisms [4]. These interactions are essential for the effective targeting and elimination of pathogens. Moreover, MPS cells contribute to tissue homeostasis and repair, processes that are vital for recovery following infection or injury [5].

The execution of distinct PCD pathways in MPS cells is governed by complex signaling cascades and molecular checkpoints. Although a detailed discussion of these regulatory mechanisms lies beyond the scope of this chapter, it is important to note that these pathways ensure the controlled induction of cell death, thereby preventing excessive inflammation and collateral tissue damage [4]. Furthermore, the regulation of these pathways is context-dependent, influenced by the tissue microenvironment and the nature of the infecting pathogen, underscoring the functional adaptability of MPS cells in diverse immunological settings [6].

In summary, this chapter focuses on the multifaceted roles of macrophages in vaccine-induced immunity, with particular emphasis on their involvement in apoptosis, necrosis, and pyroptosis. These forms of PCD are not merely consequences of immune activation but are actively exploited by vaccines to enhance immunogenicity and promote durable protection. By dissecting the interactions between vaccine platforms and macrophage biology, this section aims to elucidate the cellular and molecular mechanisms underpinning vaccine efficacy. In doing so, it contributes to the overarching objective of this book: to illuminate the diverse and dynamic roles of macrophages in health and disease. Through this lens, the text explores how macrophage-targeted strategies can be leveraged to optimize vaccine design and therapeutic innovation.

Vaccines leverage those cell-death pathways to enhance their efficacy. For example, live-attenuated vaccines activate MPS members to initiate a potent immune response, while inactivated vaccines rely on these cells to process the disarmed pathogens and present antigens effectively [2]. Subunit, recombinant, polysaccharide, and conjugate vaccines utilize MPS members to process specific pathogen components and elicit a targeted immune response [2]. Both viral vector and mRNA vaccines also depend on MPS members to process and present viral antigens, ensuring a robust immune response without the risk of causing the disease [2].

In addition to these mechanisms, adjuvants play a crucial role in enhancing vaccine efficacy by rapidly inducing chemokines and inflammatory cytokines, recruiting multiple immune cells, including the MPS members, and promoting benign apoptosis of certain innate immune cells [3]. This adjuvanticity effect is particularly beneficial in generating vaccine-specific antibodies and effector T cells, even in immunocompromised individuals. Furthermore, several cell-death pathways are essential for eliminating infected cells and regulating inflammation, thereby enhancing the overall immune response [4]. In sum, the MPS cells adapt to different immune challenges by regulating cell-death mechanisms based on the microenvironment and specific pathogens [5].

Strikingly, herbal plants have been shown to coordinate immune responses in multiple dimensions, including the modulation of apoptosis of MPS cells and the enhancement of its antioxidative activity, which can further support the efficacy of vaccines [6]. These multifaceted roles of MPS members and adjuvants underscore their importance in maintaining a robust and effective immune response, making them key players in the body's defense against infections and diseases.

Specifically, the MPS members play a crucial role in the immune response to vaccines by engaging in the clearance of senescent or dead cells, tissue repair, and the maintenance of tissue integrity and homeostasis [1, 7]. These cells are highly plastic and can adapt to various microenvironments, performing diverse functions such as antimicrobial defense, inflammation resolution, and tissue regeneration [1, 7]. The interplay between different forms of cell death in macrophages creates a coordinated and flexible system that promptly responds to the microenvironment, enhancing the overall immune response [1, 7].

Besides their crucial functions in immune response and tissue maintenance, MPS members also play a key role in regulating lipid metabolism and iron homeostasis, which are critical for their function and survival [8]. This regulation is essential for preventing the accumulation of toxic substances and ensuring the proper functioning of immune cells. For instance, natural polyphenols have been shown to modulate the activity of MPS cells, enhancing their ability to maintain immune homeostasis and respond to infections [9].

Furthermore, the interaction between MPS members and viral proteins can significantly impact the immune response. For instance, the spike protein of SARS-CoV-2 has been shown to modulate the activity of MPS cells, affecting their ability to respond to infections and maintain tissue homeostasis [10]. This interaction underscores the importance of further understanding the molecular mechanisms that govern MPS cell function and their role in immune response.

Overall, the multifaceted roles of MPS members in antigen presentation, PCD, cytokine production, and tissue repair highlight their importance in maintaining a robust and effective immune response. Their ability to adapt to various immune challenges and regulate inflammation makes them key players in the body's defense against infections and diseases. Through the diverse vaccine types and their respective PCD induction, the innate immune system, particularly the MPS members, is leveraged to provide effective protection against infectious diseases caused by pathogenic viruses, while other immunogens play a crucial role in preventing bacterial infections and their complications [2].

As previously stated, vaccines can induce cell-death patterns largely encompassing apoptosis, necrosis, and pyroptosis to combat infectious diseases, primarily through mechanisms that activate the immune system (**Table 1**). Here are some key patterns:

2. Apoptosis

This is a form of PCD where cells die in a pretty controlled manner, preventing the release of harmful substances. Most vaccines can trigger apoptosis when infecting immune cells, particularly MPS members, and then help to eliminate pathogens without causing collateral inflammation. This PCD may be split into **2.1 natural and 2.2 immunogenic** (**Table 2**). While the mechanism of natural apoptosis involves the ordinary process of PCD, the one for immunogenic apoptosis involves PCD that enhances the immune response. Concerning immune activation, natural apoptosis activates MPS members to process and present antigens, while immunogenic apoptosis stimulates MPS members to recognize and respond to pathogens.

Vaccine type	Mechanism	Target disease	Vaccine name	References
Live-Attenuated	A weakened form of the pathogen induces a strong immune response	Measles, mumps, rubella, COVID-19, MVA, yellow fever	MMR, PRIORIX, BCG, BK2102	[11–13]
Inactivated	A killed version of the pathogen induces an immune response	HAV, HBV, influenza, PV, RABV, COVID-19	Imovax, RabAvert, Havrix, Vaqta, Twinrix, IPOL, Pentacel, Pediarix, LAIV, IIV, BK2102	[14–17]
Subunit, recombinant, polysaccharide, and conjugated	Use specific pieces of the pathogen to induce a strong immune response	HBV, HPV, Hib, influenza, PCV, meningococcal	Engerix-B, Recombivax HB, Heplisav-B, Twinrix, Gardasil, Cervarix, Prevnar 13, Vaxneuvance or PCV15, Prevnar 20, Pneumovax 23, Daptacel, Infanrix, Kinrix, Pediarix, Pentacel, Quadracel, Vaxelis, ActHIB, PedvaxHIB	[13, 18]
Viral Vector	Use a modified virus to deliver genetic material that induces an immune response	COVID-19, Ebola, MVA, VSV	Vaxzevria, Covishield, Sputnik V, Convidecia, ERVEBO, Zabdeno + Mvabea, ChAdOx1 nCoV-19, Imvanex, Imvamune, Jynneos, Ervebo	[13, 19–21]
mRNA	mRNA instructs cells to produce a protein that triggers an immune response	COVID-19	Comirnaty, Spikevax	[13, 22–24]

Table 1.
Overview of certified vaccines against infectious diseases.

2.1 Licensed vaccines targeting infectious diseases and inducing natural apoptosis

2.1.1 Live-attenuated vaccines

The attenuation process often involves genetic modifications to reduce the pathogen's virulence while maintaining its ability to elicit immunity [11]. Recent advancements in genetic engineering have improved the safety and efficacy of this class of vaccines [12]. These include vaccines for diseases like measles, mumps, and rubella (MMR/PRIORIX) and TB (BCG), which activate MPS members to initiate a strong immune response [25].

2.1.2 Inactivated vaccines

This class of vaccines uses killed versions of the pathogen that causes a given disease, such as rabies (RABV; Imovax/RabAvert), hepatitis A (HAV; Havrix/Vaqta/Twinrix), and poliovirus (PV; IPOL/Pentacel/Pediarix). They usually require multiple doses to build and maintain immunity. The inactivated viruses are processed by MPS members, which present antigens to other specific cells, thereby stimulating an

Vaccine type	Natural apoptosis	Immunogenic apoptosis
Live-Attenuated	• Genetic modifications reduce pathogen virulence while preserving immunity. • Activate MPS members for a robust immune response.	• Identifies MPS members for humoral and cellular immune responses. • Evaluated in animal models showing long-term protection.
Inactivated	• Uses killed versions of pathogens. • It requires multiple doses for immunity. • Processed by MPS members to stimulate the immune response.	• Generally, it does not induce immunogenic apoptosis directly. • Indirectly contributes to immunogenic apoptosis. • Strong humoral and cellular immune responses.
Subunit, recombinant, polysaccharide, and conjugated	• Uses specific pieces of the pathogen. • Provides a targeted immune response. • Processed by MPS members.	• It does not directly induce immunogenic apoptosis. • Stimulates MPS members to recognize and respond to pathogens.
Viral Vector	• Uses replication-controlled virus as a vector. • Genetic material instructs cells to produce protein for the immune response. • Processed by MPS members.	• Might induce immunogenic apoptosis. • Enhances immune response by stimulating MPS members. • Strong cellular and humoral immune responses.
mRNA	• Uses mRNA to instruct cells to produce a protein for the immune response. • High efficacy and safety. • Processed by MPS members.	• Induces immunogenic apoptosis. • Leverages natural immune mechanisms for strong protection. • Swift development and large-scale production.

Table 2.
Comparison of two kinds of apoptosis in certified vaccines against infectious diseases.

immune response [26, 27]. Studies have shown that inactivated vaccines can effectively reduce the incidence of severe disease and maintain long-term immunity with booster doses [14, 28].

2.1.3 Subunit, recombinant, polysaccharide, and conjugate vaccines

These vaccines use specific pieces of the pathogen, such as its protein, sugar, or capsid, to elicit a targeted immune response. They provide a strong immune response targeted to key parts of the etiologic agent, such as hepatitis B (HBV; Engerix-B/Recombivax HB/Heplisav-B/Twinrix), papillomavirus (HPV; Gardasil/Cervarix), and pneumococcal (PCVs; Prevnar 13/Vaxneuvance or PCV15/Prevnar 20; and PPSV; Pneumovax 23), in which MPS members process virus-like particles and present them to other immune cells [26]. The toxoid vaccines might also be part of this category, such as diphtheria and tetanus (DTP; Daptacel/Infanrix/Kinrix/Pediarix/Pentacel/Quadracel/Vaxelis), in which MPS members process both diphtheria and tetanus toxins (plus the killed whooping cough whole bacterium) and present them to other immune cells [26].

2.1.4 Viral vector vaccines

This class of vaccines uses a replication-controlled virus as a vector to deliver genetic material from the pathogen that causes the given disease, such as for COVID-19 (Vaxzevria/Covishield/Sputnik V/Convidecia) and Ebola (ERVEBO/Zabdeno + Mvabea). This genetic material instructs cells to produce a protein that triggers an immune response. The MPS members play a role in processing and presenting the viral antigens [26]. Viral vectors can induce strong cellular and humoral immune responses, often without the need for adjuvants [20, 29].

2.1.5 mRNA vaccines

These vaccines, such as for COVID-19 (Comirnaty/Spikevax), the MPS members help process the spike protein of SARS-CoV-2 produced by cells and present it to T cells using mRNA to instruct cells to produce a protein that triggers an immune response. This class of vaccines does not contain live organisms, so there is no risk of causing the disease [26]. The mRNA vaccines have shown high efficacy and safety, with rapid development and scalability [14, 29].

2.2 Licensed vaccines targeting infectious diseases and inducing immunogenic apoptosis

2.2.1 Live-attenuated vaccines

These include immunogens for diseases like COVID-19 (BK2102). This vaccine candidate has shown promising results targeting the MPS members for later inducing humoral and cellular immune responses without significant tissue damage. It has been tested in animal models and has demonstrated long-term protection [12].

2.2.2 Inactivated vaccines

These vaccines generally do not induce immunogenic apoptosis directly. Instead, they work by stimulating the immune system to recognize and respond to the antigens present in the vaccine. However, there are some instances where inactivated vaccines can indirectly contribute to immunogenic apoptosis, aiding MPS members in clearing infected cells. These include influenza (LAIV and IIV) and SARS-CoV-2 (BK2102) vaccines, which are known to induce strong humoral and cellular immune responses, including immunogenic apoptosis, which are crucial for effective, protective immunity [14, 28, 30].

2.2.3 Subunit, recombinant, polysaccharide, and conjugate vaccines

Once again, while this class of vaccines does not directly induce immunogenic apoptosis, they are highly effective in stimulating the MPS members to help recognize and respond to specific pathogens [31]. These include HBV (Engerix-B/Recombivax HB), HPV (Gardasil/Cervarix), *Haemophilus influenzae* type b (Hib; ActHIB/PedvaxHIB), and the PCV (Prevnar 13/Vaxneuvance/Prevnar 20/Pneumovax 23).

2.2.4 Viral vector vaccines

These vaccines might indeed induce immunogenic apoptosis, enhancing the immune response by first stimulating the MPS members. For instance, the COVID-19 (ChAdOx1 nCoV-19), smallpox (MVA; Imvanex/Imvamune/Jynneos), and VSV (Ervebo) vaccines are a few platforms to be used for this end [30, 32]. Viral vectors are advantageous due to their ability to elicit strong cellular and humoral immune responses [20, 29].

2.2.5 mRNA vaccines

These vaccines have shown promising results in inducing immunogenic apoptosis, which enhances the immune response. A promising technology for COVID-19 (Comirnaty/Spikevax) is able to leverage the natural immune mechanisms triggered by the MPS members to provide strong and long-lasting protection [33]. The technology used in mRNA vaccines enables swift development and large-scale production, positioning them as a highly effective tool in contemporary vaccinology [34].

3. Necrosis

This is an uncontrolled form of cell death that often results in inflammation (**Figure 2**). Some vaccines can induce necrosis to alert the immune system to the presence of an infection. Though very few vaccines have been associated with inducing necrosis, particularly among MPS members, this is not a common or intended effect.

3.1 Licensed vaccines targeting infectious diseases and inducing necrosis

3.1.1 Live-attenuated vaccines

This class of vaccines is generally designed to be safe and effective, very rarely inducing cell necrosis, particularly in individuals with compromised immune system.

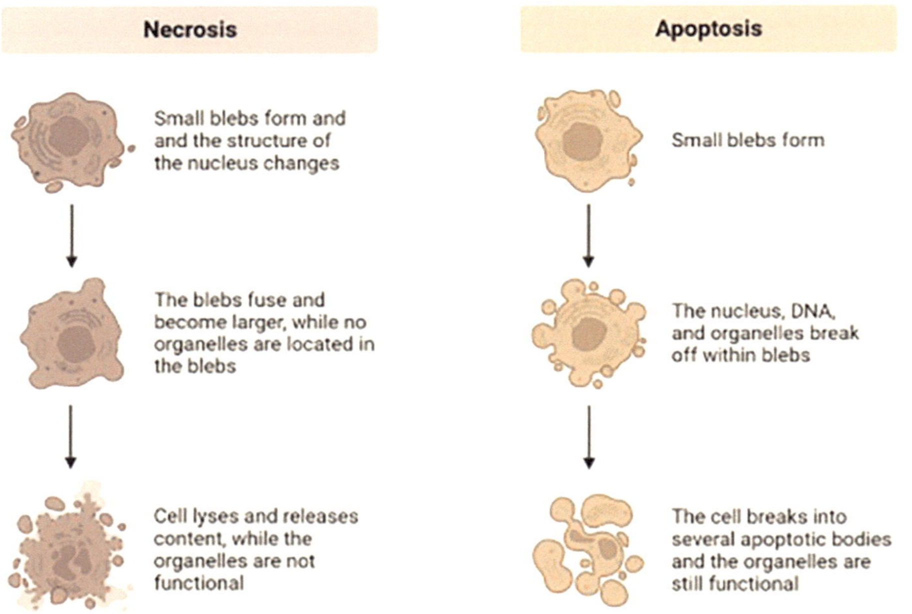

Figure 2.
Comparison of the main processes for necrosis vs. apoptosis in immune cells. Adapted from a BioRender template.

These include vaccines for diseases like measles, mumps, and rubella (MMR II) that are generally safe, but there have been rare instances of severe inflammatory responses that could lead to cell necrosis [11] Also, for yellow fever (YF-VAX), the vaccine might cause severe reactions, including viscerotropic disease, which may involve necrosis of the MPS members [35], and for MVA (ACAM2000), the vaccine induces necrosis at the site of inoculation, especially in immunocompromised individuals [35].

3.1.2 Inactivated vaccines

These vaccines use destroyed versions of the pathogen, such as RABV (RabAvert), where severe local reactions have been reported, which can include cell necrosis [36], IPV (IPOL), that in rare cases, significant limited adverse events may occur, potentially leading to cell necrosis [36], and influenza (Fluzone), where there have been rare reports of severe inflammatory responses that could lead to necrosis of MPS members [37].

3.1.3 Subunit, recombinant, polysaccharide, and conjugate vaccines

While it is very unusual, a few of those vaccines may induce cell necrosis, particularly in individuals with compromised immune systems or underlying health conditions. Examples are HBV (Engerix-B) with intense localized responses including cell necrosis [11], HPV (Gardasil), embracing rare instances of severe inflammatory responses that could lead to necrosis of MPS members [38], PCV (Prevnar 13), including pronounced site-specific reactions [31], and meningococcal (Menactra) quite rarely accompanying severe local inflammatory responses potentially leading to cell necrosis [39].

3.1.4 Viral vector vaccines

This class of immunogens employs a virus with controlled replication as a vector to introduce genetic material from the pathogen responsible for the disease, such as for Ebola (Ervebo), which uses an rVSV as a vector to express the Ebola virus glycoprotein. Studies indicate that this immunogen may induce cell necrosis in certain contexts [40]. The COVID-19 vaccine (Ad26.COV2.S or Jcovden) employs an rAd26 vector to express the SARS-CoV-2 spike protein. A few studies have reported inflammatory responses that could lead to cell necrosis of MPS members [32]. Finally, the MVA vaccine (ACAM2000) is a highly attenuated vaccinia virus strain. Trials have shown that it may induce cell necrosis under certain conditions [33].

3.1.5 mRNA vaccines

Once again, and due to their nature, those single vaccines target the SARS-CoV-2 only and have been associated with inducing necrosis of MPS members. These vaccines for COVID-19 (BNT162b2/mRNA-1273) are currently widely used, and studies have shown that they might induce acute local inflammation [33, 34].

4. Pyroptosis

This is a highly inflammatory form of PCD, often triggered by infections (**Figure 3**). It helps to release inflammatory signals that recruit immune cells, mostly

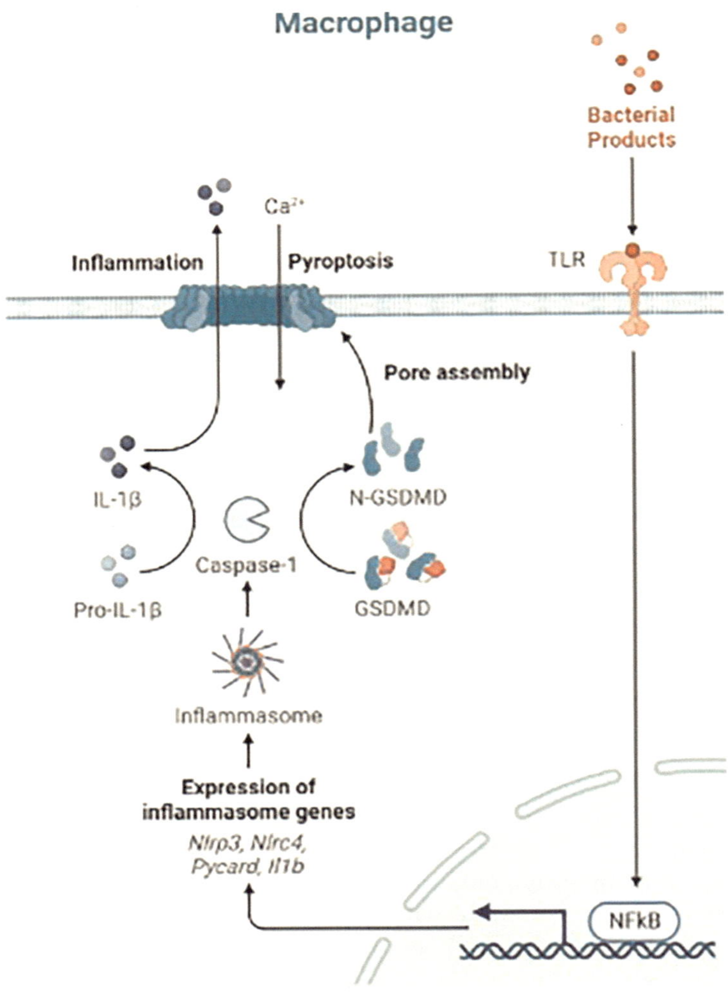

Figure 3.
Pyroptosis in an MPS member (e.g., macrophage): Main inflammatory mechanisms and pathways. Adapted from a BioRender template.

MPS members, to the site of infection. The majority of research on pyroptosis currently focuses on its role in the immune response to natural infections rather than vaccine-induced responses.

4.1 Licensed vaccines targeting infectious diseases and inducing pyroptosis

4.1.1 Live-attenuated vaccines

While this class of vaccines is known to induce strong immune responses, specific evidence linking these immunogens to the induction of pyroptosis is limited. Currently, there are no specific experimental or licensed vaccines in this category that have been documented to induce pyroptosis.

4.1.2 Inactivated vaccines

These vaccines use inactive forms of the pathogen, such as influenza (Fluzone/Flucelvax), where vaccine research has indicated a fairly induction of pyroptosis in MPS members through the activation of the NLRP3 inflammasome [41]. Similarly, studies on the HBV (Engerix-B/Heplisav-B) have shown triggering of pyroptosis in hepatocytes via the AIM2 inflammasome [42].

4.1.3 Subunit, recombinant, polysaccharide, and conjugate vaccines

This class of vaccines leverages the inflammatory nature of pyroptosis to enhance immune responses, making them promising candidates for immunotherapy. Examples are HBV (Engerix-B), a subunit that has been shown to induce pyroptosis in hepatocytes via the AIM2 inflammasome [43], the PCV (PPSV23), where a study has indicated that polysaccharide nanofiber-stabilized microparticles may induce pyroptosis in liver cells [44], and Hib (OMPC), a complex comprising the outer membrane in a conjugated vaccine, engaging human Toll-like receptor 2 in a MyD88-dependent manner, leading to cytokine production and immune responses [45]. The activation of TLR2 can trigger inflammasome pathways, potentially leading to the induction of pyroptosis in MPS members like dendritic cells [41].

4.1.4 Viral vector vaccines

These vaccines utilize a replication-limited virus as a carrier to introduce genetic material from the pathogen responsible for the disease, such as for COVID-19 (Vaxzevria/Ad26.COV2.S or Jcovden). Once again, the MPS members play a role in processing and presenting the SARS-CoV-2 antigens [26]. Those are adenovirus-vectored vaccines shown to induce pyroptosis in MPS members through the activation of the NLRP3 inflammasome [20, 41].

4.1.5 mRNA vaccines

Currently, there is limited evidence directly linking licensed mRNA vaccines to the induction of pyroptosis. In these immunogens, such as for COVID-19 (Comirnaty/Spikevax), the MPS members help process the spike protein of SARS-CoV-2 produced by cells and present it to T cells using mRNA to instruct cells to produce a protein that triggers an immune response. Besides, those most well-known licensed mRNA vaccines have not been specifically documented to induce pyroptosis [34, 46].

> The field of BCG vaccine research has significant potential for advancement, particularly in understanding its immunological effects and applications. Dr. Paulo Antas has extensively studied the BCG Moreau strain, which has demonstrated a superior ability to induce inflammatory cytokine profiles compared to other strains. This strain has been shown to upregulate crucial immune markers on human monocytes, thereby enhancing the body's immune response. Dr. Antas has focused primarily on the mechanisms of cell death and inflammatory responses triggered by BCG infection. His studies have revealed that the BCG Moreau strain induces caspase-1 expression and dependent cell death, underscoring the importance of cell integrity in the immune response to BCG vaccination. These findings are vital for understanding how the immune system interacts with mycobacterial antigens and controlling infections. Furthermore, Dr. Antas' research suggests

that revamping the BCG revaccination strategy could be beneficial. By leveraging the unique properties of the BCG Moreau strain, it is possible to boost immune responses more effectively. Overall, Dr. Antas' work has provided valuable insights into the immunomodulatory effects of the BCG vaccine, paving the way for improved vaccination strategies and therapeutic approaches in the fight against tuberculosis.

5. Conclusions

These classes of vaccines leverage the innate immune system, particularly the MPS, to provide effective protection against infectious diseases caused by pathogenic viruses. Other immunogens are crucial in preventing bacterial infections and their complications.

Understanding the mechanisms of apoptosis, necrosis, and pyroptosis is crucial in the development and optimization of vaccines. Each of these processes plays a unique role in the immune response, influencing the efficacy and safety of various vaccine types. As such, apoptosis is the prototypic PCD that allows for the controlled elimination of infected or damaged cells without causing inflammation. This process is essential for maintaining tissue homeostasis and ensuring that the immune system can effectively respond to pathogens without causing collateral damage. Conversely, necrosis is an uncontrolled form of cell death that often results from severe injury or infection. While necrosis can lead to inflammation and tissue damage, understanding its triggers and effects is vital for improving vaccine formulations to minimize adverse reactions, especially in individuals with compromised immune systems. Finally, pyroptosis is an inflammatory form of PCD that plays a significant role in the immune response by eliminating infected cells and alerting the immune system to the presence of pathogens. Leveraging pyroptosis in vaccine design can enhance immune responses, making vaccines more effective in combating diseases.

The interplay between these cell-death mechanisms and vaccine-induced immune responses underscores the importance of continued research and innovation in vaccinology. By harnessing the beneficial aspects of apoptosis and pyroptosis while mitigating the risks associated with necrosis, studies and trials might be developed to be safer and deemed to uncover aspects for more effective vaccines. This knowledge not only advances our understanding of immunology but also paves the way for the creation of the next generation of vaccines against infectious diseases that offer robust protection with minimal side effects.

In sum, the intricate balance between apoptosis, necrosis, and pyroptosis is a cornerstone of vaccine development. As we continue to explore and refine these processes, we move closer to achieving optimal vaccine efficacy and safety, ultimately contributing to better public health outcomes worldwide.

Author details

Paulo R.Z. Antas[1,2]

1 Oswaldo Cruz Institute, Fiocruz, Brazil

2 Federal University of Ceará, Brazil

*Address all correspondence to: paulo.zuquim@fiocruz.br

References

[1] Makuch M, Stepanechko M, Bzowska M. The dance of macrophage death: The interplay between the inevitable and the microenvironment. Frontiers in Immunology. 2024;**15**: 1330461

[2] Chekaoui A, Garofalo M, Gad B, Staniszewska M, Chiaro J, Pancer K, et al. Cancer vaccines: An update on recent achievements and prospects for cancer therapy. Clinical and Experimental Medicine. 2024;**25**(1):24

[3] Ko EJ, Kang SM. Immunology and efficacy of MF59-adjuvanted vaccines. Human Vaccines & Immunotherapeutics. 2018;**14**(12): 3041-3045

[4] Silva MJA, Ribeiro LR, Lima KVB, Lima LNGC. Adaptive immunity to SARS-CoV-2 infection: A systematic review. Frontiers in Immunology. 2022; **13**:1001198

[5] Hampel B, Fortschegger K, Ressler S, Chang MW, Unterluggauer H, Breitwieser A, et al. Increased expression of extracellular proteins as a hallmark of human endothelial cell in vitro senescence. Experimental Gerontology. 2006;**41**(5):474-481

[6] Zhang Y, Li Y, Wang X, Qu R, Li J, Li T, et al. Herbal plants coordinate COVID-19 in multiple dimensions—An insight analysis for clinically applied remedies. International Journal of Medical Sciences. 2020;**17**(18):3125-3145

[7] Zhou Y, Wei Y, Tian X, Wei X. Cancer vaccines: Current status and future directions. Journal of Hematology & Oncology. 2025;**18**(1):18

[8] Bah SY, Dickinson P, Forster T, Kampmann B, Ghazal P. Immune oxysterols: Role in mycobacterial infection and inflammation. The Journal of Steroid Biochemistry and Molecular Biology. 2017;**169**:152-163

[9] Bernini R, Velotti F. Natural polyphenols as immunomodulators to rescue immune response homeostasis: Quercetin as a research model against severe COVID-19. Molecules. 2021;**26**(19):5803

[10] Miltner N, Linkner TR, Ambrus V, Al-Muffti AS, Ahmad H, Mótyán JA, et al. Early suppression of antiviral host response and protocadherins by SARS-CoV-2 spike protein in THP-1-derived macrophage-like cells. Frontiers in Immunology. 2022;**13**:999233

[11] Antia R, Ahmed H, Bull JJ. Directed attenuation to enhance vaccine immunity. PLoS Computational Biology. 2021;**17**(2):e1008602

[12] Suzuki, Okutani M, Okamura S, Gis T, Sasaki H, Lee S, Kashiwabara A, et al. Immunogenicity and safety of a live-attenuated SARS-CoV-2 vaccine candidate based on multiple attenuation mechanisms. eLife. 11 Feb 2025;**13**: RP97532

[13] Montico B, Nigro A, Casolaro V, Dal Col J. Immunogenic apoptosis as a novel tool for anticancer vaccine development. International Journal of Molecular Sciences. 2018;**19**(2):594

[14] Xu S, Li J, Wang H, Wang F, Yin Z, Wang Z. Real-world effectiveness and factors associated with effectiveness of inactivated SARS-CoV-2 vaccines: A systematic review and meta-regression analysis. BMC Medicine. 2023;**21**(1):160

[15] Sanders BP, Liu Y, Brandjes A, van Hoek V, Oakes d LR I, Lewis J, et al.

Brunenders: A partially attenuated historic poliovirus type I vaccine strain. The Journal of General Virology. 2015; **96**(9):2614-2622

[16] Khoshnood S, Arshadi M, Akrami S, Koupaei M, Ghahramanpour H, Shariati A, et al. An overview on inactivated and live-attenuated SARS-CoV-2 vaccines. Journal of Clinical Laboratory Analysis. 2022;**36**(5):e24418

[17] Corripio-Miyar Y, MacLeod CL, Mair I, Mellanby RJ, Moore BD, McNeilly TN. Self-adjuvanting calcium-phosphate-coated microcrystal-based vaccines induce pyroptosis in human and livestock immune cells. Vaccines (Basel). 2023;**11**(7):1229

[18] Wang Y, Liu H, Wang B, Gheyret G, Qin J, Wang H, et al. Recent advances in the biosynthesis of polysaccharide-based antimicrobial glycoconjugate vaccines. Frontiers in Microbiology. 2024;**15**: 1457908

[19] Deng S, Liang H, Chen P, Li Y, Li Z, Fan S, et al. Viral vector vaccine development and application during the COVID-19 pandemic. Microorganisms. 2022;**10**(7):1450

[20] Travieso T, Li J, Mahesh S, Mello JDFR, Blasi M. The use of viral vectors in vaccine development. npj Vaccines. 2022;**7**(1):75

[21] Li YD, Chi WY, Su JH, Ferrall L, Hung CF, Wu TC. Coronavirus vaccine development: From SARS and MERS to COVID-19. Journal of Biomedical Science. 2020;**27**(1):104

[22] Leong KY, Tham SK, Poh CL. Revolutionizing immunization: A comprehensive review of mRNA vaccine technology and applications. Virology Journal. 2025;**22**(1):71

[23] Wang YS, Kumari M, Chen GH, Hong MH, Yuan JP, Tsai JL, et al. mRNA-based vaccines and therapeutics: An in-depth survey of current and upcoming clinical applications. Journal of Biomedical Science. 2023; **30**(1):84

[24] Gote V, Bolla PK, Kommineni N, Butreddy A, Nukala PK, Palakurthi SS, et al. A comprehensive review of mRNA vaccines. International Journal of Molecular Sciences. 2023;**24**(3):2700

[25] Brancewicz J, Wójcik N, Sarnowska Z, Robak J, Król M. The multifaceted role of macrophages in biology and diseases. International Journal of Molecular Sciences. 2025;**26**(5):2107

[26] Agrawal A, Weinberger B. Editorial: The impact of immunosenescence and senescence of immune cells on responses to infection and vaccination. Frontiers in Aging. 2022;**3**:882494

[27] Lytle AG, Shen S, McGettigan JP. Lymph node but not intradermal injection site macrophages are critical for germinal center formation and antibody responses to rabies vaccination. Journal of Virology. 2015; **89**(5):2842-2848

[28] Xia S, Duan K, Zhang Y, Zhao D, Zhang H, Xie Z, et al. Effect of an inactivated vaccine against SARS-CoV-2 on safety and immunogenicity outcomes: Interim analysis of 2 randomized clinical trials. JAMA. 2020;**324**(10):951-960

[29] Parish LA, Rele S, Hofmeyer KA, Luck BB, Wolfe DN. Strategic and technical considerations in manufacturing viral vector vaccines for the biomedical advanced research and development authority threats. Vaccines (Basel). 2025;**13**(1):73

[30] Hajra D, Datey A, Chakravortty D. Attenuation methods for live vaccines.

Methods in Molecular Biology. 2021; **2183**:331-356

[31] Guo M, Guo X, Zhang C, Zhu S, Zhang Y, Gu T, et al. Novel pneumococcal protein-polysaccharide conjugate vaccine based on biotin-streptavidin. Infection and Immunity. 2022;**90**(1):e0035221

[32] Lauer KB, Borrow R, Blanchard TJ. Multivalent and multipathogen viral vector vaccines. Clinical and Vaccine Immunology. 2017; **24**(1):e00298-16

[33] Ahn JH, Lee J, Roh G, Lee NY, Bae HJ, Kwon E, et al. Impact of administration routes and dose frequency on the toxicology of SARS-CoV-2 mRNA vaccines in mice model. Archives of Toxicology. 2025;**99**(2): 755-773

[34] Zhou F, Wang M, Wang Z, Li W, Lu X. Screening of novel tumor-associated antigens for lung adenocarcinoma mRNA vaccine development based on pyroptosis phenotype genes. BMC Cancer. 2024; **24**(1):28

[35] Zeng R, Pan W, Lin Y, Liang M, Fu J, Weng S, et al. A safe and efficient double-gene-deleted live attenuated immersion vaccine to prevent the disease caused by the infectious spleen and kidney necrosis virus. Journal of Virology. 2023;**97**(7):e0085723

[36] Walsh G. Biopharmaceutical benchmarks 2018. Nature Biotechnology. 2018;**36**(12):1136-1145

[37] Orenstein WA, Plotkin S. Providing MMR vaccine to children. Minnesota Medicine. 1991;**74**(3):7-8

[38] Rappuoli R. Glycoconjugate vaccines: Principles and mechanisms. Science Translational Medicine. 2018;**10**(456): eaat4615

[39] Gupta S, Pellett S. Recent developments in vaccine design: From live vaccines to recombinant toxin vaccines. Toxins (Basel). 2023;**15**(9):563

[40] O'Connell CM, Jasperse B, Hagen CJ, Titong A, Verardi PH. Replication-inducible vaccinia virus vectors with enhanced safety in vivo. PLoS One. 2020;**15**(4):e0230711

[41] He S, Li L, Chen H, Hu X, Wang W, Zhang H, et al. PRRSV infection induces gasdermin D-driven pyroptosis of porcine alveolar macrophages through NLRP3 inflammasome activation. Journal of Virology. 2022;**96**(14): e0212721

[42] Zhang DX, Liu BY, Xue FF, Tang YL, Yan MJ, Wang SX, et al. Paclobutrazol induces triterpenoid biosynthesis via downregulation of the negative transcriptional regulator SlMYB in sanghuangporus lonicericola. Communications Biology. 2025;**8**(1):551

[43] Xie WH, Ding J, Xie XX, Yang XH, Wu XF, Chen ZX, et al. Hepatitis B virus X protein promotes liver cell pyroptosis under oxidative stress through NLRP3 inflammasome activation. Inflammation Research. 2020;**69**(7):683-696

[44] Li Q, Hatakeyama M, Kitaoka T. Polysaccharide nanofiber-stabilized Pickering emulsion microparticles induce pyroptotic cell death in hepatocytes and Kupffer cells. Small. 2023;**19**(27):e2207433

[45] Latz E, Franko J, Golenbock DT, Schreiber JR. Haemophilus influenzae type b-outer membrane protein complex glycoconjugate vaccine induces cytokine production by engaging human toll-like receptor 2 (TLR2) and requires the

presence of TLR2 for optimal immunogenicity. Journal of Immunology. 2004;**172**(4):2431-2438

[46] Lin Q, Liang L, Wang Q, Wang X, You Y, Rong Y, et al. Identification of novel tumor pyroptosis-related antigens and pyroptosis subtypes for developing mRNA vaccines in pancreatic adenocarcinoma. Biomedicine. 2024;**12**(4):726

Section 4

Autophagy in Macrophages

Chapter 4

Autophagy in Macrophages: Physiological Guardians and Pathological Biomarkers in Health and Disease

Jiexing Tan, Changsheng He and Li Gong

Abstract

Macrophages, as pivotal sentinels of the immune system, rely on autophagy to maintain cellular homeostasis, modulate immune responses, and adapt to dynamic microenvironments. This chapter investigates the twofold function of autophagy in macrophages, with a focus on its essential roles in the physiological processes of tissue restoration, pathogen clearance, and metabolic regulation, alongside its pathological implications in chronic inflammation, autoimmune disorders, cancer, and infectious diseases. We dissect the molecular machinery of autophagy—including ATG proteins, mTOR/AMPK signaling, and lysosomal pathways—and their integration with macrophage polarization (M1/M2 phenotypes) and immunometabolic reprogramming. Key biomarkers of autophagic flux, such as LC3-II, p62/SQSTM1, and LAMP-1, are evaluated for their diagnostic and prognostic utility in diseases such as atherosclerosis, sepsis, and rheumatoid arthritis. Furthermore, we highlight emerging therapeutic strategies targeting macrophage autophagy, such as pharmacological enhancers (e.g., rapamycin) and inhibitors (e.g., chloroquine), while addressing challenges in translating these approaches due to context-dependent outcomes and off-target effects. By bridging mechanistic insights with clinical relevance, this chapter underscores autophagy as a dynamic interface between macrophage physiology and pathology, offering novel avenues for biomarker discovery and precision medicine.

Keywords: autophagy, macrophages, biomarkers, immunometabolism, inflammation, disease pathogenesis, therapeutic targeting, lysosomal degradation, cellular homeostasis, regulatory mechanisms

1. Introduction

As an evolutionarily conserved quality control system, autophagy serves as a crucial mechanism for cellular homeostasis through its capacity to eliminate damaged organelles, misfolded proteins, and invasive pathogens. Within macrophages—versatile sentinel cells bridging innate and adaptive immunity—this self-digestive process undergoes sophisticated regulation, profoundly influencing their functional

IntechOpen

adaptability. Current classifications delineate three principal autophagic subtypes: macroautophagy, mitophagy, and chaperone-mediated autophagy (CMA), each exhibiting unique molecular signatures and physiological consequences [1–3].

Classic macroautophagy begins when unique double-membrane autophagosomes are generated. These autophagosomes sequester cytoplasmic elements and eventually combine with lysosomes, triggering the breakdown of their enclosed substances. A group of evolutionarily preserved autophagy-related (ATG) proteins governs this sequential process. Significantly, the lipid modification of LC3, where cytosolic LC3-I is transformed into membrane-anchored LC3-II, marks the completion of autophagosome maturation [4]. Beyond its fundamental role in cellular housekeeping, macrophage macroautophagy demonstrates immunomodulatory prowess through dual functionality: sustaining metabolic demands under stress while orchestrating immune responses *via* antigen processing and microbial clearance. Mitophagy represents a specialized quality control mechanism that selectively removes compromised mitochondria through receptor-mediated recognition systems, including the PINK1/Parkin axis and NIX/BNIP3 pathways. By eliminating mitochondria prone to generating reactive oxygen species (mtROS), this selective autophagy subtype in macrophages exerts anti-inflammatory effects through suppression of NLRP3 inflammasome activation, a critical checkpoint in inflammation resolution [5, 6]. Distinguished from vesicle-dependent pathways, CMA employs a precise substrate recognition system where cytosolic HSC70 chaperones identify proteins containing KFERQ-targeting motifs, facilitating their lysosomal translocation through LAMP2A receptor complexes. Emerging evidence suggests macrophage CMA not only maintains proteomic equilibrium but also modulates inflammatory cascades through controlled degradation of regulatory enzymes and transcriptional activators [3].

2. Interplay between autophagic machinery and macrophage functional dynamics (phagocytosis, cytokine secretion)

The intricate dialog between autophagy and macrophage effector functions operates through multiple molecular circuits. Mechanistically, this interplay manifests most prominently in phagocytic processes—the sentinel function of these immune sentinels. Autophagic membranes dynamically contribute to phagosome biogenesis, with nascent autophagosomes providing lipid bilayers that accelerate phagocytic cup formation during microbial engulfment. Core autophagy machinery components, including ATG5 and Beclin-1, facilitate phagolysosome maturation through membrane remodeling, thereby optimizing intracellular pathogen destruction. Conversely, genetic ablation of autophagy pathways compromises efferocytosis (the clearance of apoptotic cells), resulting in cellular debris accumulation that triggers necroinflammation—a hallmark of chronic inflammatory disorders [5–7].

The regulatory influence of autophagy extends to cytokine networks through dual modulation mechanisms. In terms of protein stability, selective autophagic degradation of pro-interleukin-1β precursors and direct inhibition of NLRP3 inflammasome assembly serve as critical brakes on excessive inflammatory responses. Paradoxically, autophagy simultaneously enables anti-inflammatory programming through mitochondrial quality control in alternatively activated macrophages. By eliminating ROS-generating mitochondria *via* mitophagy, this process preserves metabolic flexibility required for IL-10 production during tissue repair phases. Emerging studies reveal autophagy's role as a metabolic integrator, interfacing with glycolytic flux and oxidative phosphorylation to dictate macrophage polarization states. This energy sensor function ultimately determines whether macrophages adopt pro-inflammatory M1 phenotypes or transition towards wound-healing M2 phenotypes [8, 9].

Autophagy in macrophages acts as a variable resistor, balancing immune activation and degradation. Dysregulation of autophagy can lead to chronic inflammation, autoimmune diseases, and impaired host defense, highlighting its therapeutic potential in macrophage centric diseases.

2.1 The physiological functions of autophagy in macrophages

Autophagy, a crucial cellular mechanism, plays a pivotal role in determining the functionality of macrophages in multiple physiological scenarios. Through regulating the renewal of cellular substances and modulating immune activities, autophagy enables macrophages to maintain tissue equilibrium, resist microbial invasions, and contribute to tissue restoration. In the following sections, we will discuss the major physiological functions of autophagy in macrophages in detail.

2.2 Homeostasis: Clearance of damaged organelles and proteins

Macrophages operate in dynamic environments where they encounter oxidative stress, metabolic byproducts, and damaged organelles. Autophagy serves as a quality control mechanism by selectively degrading dysfunctional mitochondria (mitophagy), endoplasmic reticulum (reticulophagy), and aggregated proteins. For instance, mitophagy in macrophages is driven by the PINK1/Parkin pathway or hypoxia-induced receptors like FUNDC1, which tags depolarized mitochondria for autophagosomal engulfment [2]. Defective mitophagy leads to mitochondrial dysfunction, contributing to Parkinson's disease pathology through ROS accumulation and neuronal death [10]. Moreover, mitophagy prevents inflammation by clearing mitochondrial DNA (mtDNA). In aged macrophages, impaired mitophagy results in cytosolic mtDNA leakage, activating the cGAS-STING pathway and driving sterile inflammation in liver injury [11]. Parkin and PINK1 further suppress STING signaling by removing damaged mitochondria, highlighting mitophagy's anti-inflammatory role [10].

Inability to clear impaired mitochondria leads to mitochondrial reactive oxygen species (mtROS) accumulation. This subsequent mtROS accumulation initiates the activation of the NLRP3 inflammasome, prompting an overabundant release of pro-inflammatory cytokines, including IL-1β and IL-18. Analogously, chaperone-mediated autophagy (CMA) selectively degrades oxidized or malformed proteins, such as SOD1 and IκBα. Through this process, CMA averts proteotoxic stress, thus safeguarding cellular integrity.

By preserving organelle and proteome health, autophagy enables macrophages to sustain their functional capacity under homeostatic and stress conditions [3, 12]. CMA deficiency in macrophages promotes lipid accumulation, linking CMA dysfunction to metabolic disorders such as atherosclerosis [13]. As a pivotal lysosomal stress adaptation pathway, the TFEB-GDF15 axis combats obesity and insulin insensitivity by boosting autophagic activity and accelerating lipid breakdown [14]. Autophagy proteins restrict NLRP3 inflammasome activation by sequestering mtDNA and preventing its interaction with NLRP3. Conversely, defective autophagy in aging or disease exacerbates mtDNA-driven inflammation, underscoring the delicate balance between mitochondrial clearance and immune activation [15].

2.3 Antimicrobial defense: Xenophagy in pathogen elimination

Autophagy contributes significantly to innate immunity *via* xenophagy, a specific autophagic process. Xenophagy selectively eliminates intracellular pathogens, including bacteria, viruses, and parasites, directly bolstering the body's first-line defense mechanisms. Upon pathogen recognition *via* pattern recognition receptors (PRRs), macrophages initiate xenophagy by recruiting autophagy machinery (e.g., LC3, ATG5) to pathogen-containing vacuoles or cytosolic invaders. For example: autophagosomes engulf *Mycobacterium tuberculosis* and subsequently merge with lysosomes, triggering the bacterium's degradation process. *Salmonella* Typhimurium escaping into the cytosol is tagged with ubiquitin, recruiting autophagy adaptors (e.g., p62/SQSTM1, NDP52) for autophagic destruction. Autophagy also enhances antimicrobial activity by delivering pathogen-derived antigens to MHC-II compartments, bridging innate and adaptive immunity. Furthermore, autophagy-related proteins like ATG12-ATG5 conjugate inhibit inflammasome hyperactivation, preventing collateral tissue damage during infection [4, 8, 16, 17]. Pathogens exploit autophagy to evade immune detection. For example, *M. tuberculosis* inhibits mitophagy to sustain intracellular survival, yet paradoxically, mitophagy-deficient macrophages mount stronger antimicrobial responses *via* unfolded protein response (UPR) pathways [18]. SARS-CoV-2 disrupts iron metabolism, elevating ROS and impairing autophagic clearance, which compromises antiviral immunity [19]. Therapeutic interventions, such as zinc oxide nanoparticles, exhibit biphasic effects—inducing ROS-dependent autophagy to inhibit Mycobacterium at low doses while causing cytotoxicity at higher concentrations [19].

2.4 Tissue repair: Resolution of inflammation and M2 polarization

Autophagy extends its function beyond pathogen elimination, playing a pivotal role in inflammation resolution and promoting tissue repair. When macrophages undergo a phenotypic shift from pro-inflammatory M1 to anti-inflammatory and reparative M2, autophagy is instrumental in orchestrating metabolic reprogramming. M2 macrophages primarily utilize oxidative phosphorylation (OXPHOS) and fatty acid oxidation (FAO). These metabolic pathways are maintained by autophagy, which regulate mitochondrial quality control and facilitate the turnover of lipid droplets. For instance: Autophagy clears damaged mitochondria in M2 macrophages, reducing mtROS and NLRP3 inflammasome activity. Lysosomal degradation of lipid droplets *via* lipophagy provides free fatty acids to fuel FAO, a metabolic hallmark of M2 macrophages. Autophagy also enhances antimicrobial activity by delivering pathogen-derived antigens to MHC-II compartments, bridging innate and adaptive immunity. Furthermore, Autophagy also promotes efferocytosis (clearance of apoptotic cells) by enhancing lysosomal acidification and degrading engulfed cellular debris. This prevents secondary necrosis and the release of pro-inflammatory damage-associated molecular patterns (DAMPs). Additionally, autophagy acts as a crucial regulator by curbing the overproduction of pro-inflammatory cytokines such as IL-1β and TNF-α, while simultaneously boosting the secretion of anti-inflammatory factors including IL-10 and TGF-β. This dynamic equilibrium fosters a microenvironment ideal for tissue remodeling, as evidenced by studies [9, 19, 20]. Moreover, autophagy is pivotal in the transformation of pro-inflammatory M1 macrophages into their anti-inflammatory M2 counterparts. A case in point is USP19, which accelerates the autophagy-mediated degradation of the NLRP3 inflammasome. This process inhibits IL-1β release, thereby facilitating the polarization toward the M2 phenotype [21]. Metabolic reprogramming is central to this process: Succinate dehydrogenase activity fuels M1 inflammatory responses [22], while autophagy supports fatty acid oxidation to drive M2 polarization [23]. The Nrf2 pathway, a master regulator of antioxidant responses, collaborates with autophagy to mitigate tissue injury. Nrf2 deficiency exacerbates sepsis-induced lung damage by dysregulating autophagy-dependent NF-κB/PPARγ signaling, impairing M2 polarization [23].

3. Autophagy dysregulation as a pathological biomarker: Insights into chronic inflammation, cancer, and neurodegeneration

Autophagy, while essential for cellular homeostasis, becomes a double-edged sword when dysregulated. Emerging evidence highlights autophagy dysfunction as a critical pathological biomarker across diverse diseases, reflecting its role in driving chronic inflammation, tumor progression, and neurodegenerative pathology. Below, we discuss how impaired autophagy in macrophages contributes to these disease states. Understanding these mechanisms provides insights into potential therapeutic strategies targeting autophagy for disease treatment.

3.1 Chronic inflammatory diseases: NLRP3 inflammasome activation

Inflammasomes, especially the NLRP3 inflammasome, are essential components of the innate immune system, responding to pathogens and cellular stressors [24, 25]. Nevertheless, uncontrolled activation of the NLRP3 inflammasome is the characteristic of numerous chronic inflammatory disorders. Mitochondrial impairment is central to NLRP3 inflammasome activation; when mitochondria are damaged, they release reactive oxygen species (ROS) and mitochondrial DNA. These substances initiate the process of inflammasome assembly [26].

The process of autophagy, particularly mitophagy—the targeted elimination of damaged mitochondria—is fundamental for preserving mitochondrial integrity and preventing excessive activation of the NLRP3 inflammasome [27]. Genetic abnormalities in autophagy-related genes, including Atg16l1, can disrupt mitophagy. As Saitoh et al. reported, the absence of Atg16L1 increases endotoxin-induced IL-1β production, underscoring autophagy's pivotal role in modulating the NLRP3 inflammasome [28]. Autophagy also directly engages with inflammasome components. Proteins associated with autophagy often function to suppress inflammasome activation. When autophagic processes malfunction, these regulatory mechanisms break down, leading to unregulated secretion of pro-inflammatory cytokines such as IL-1β and IL-18. This cytokine overproduction contributes to the chronic inflammation observed in conditions like atherosclerosis. Qiao et al. found that impaired chaperone-mediated autophagy exacerbates inflammation and atherosclerosis by promoting NLRP3 inflammasome activation [29]. Recent findings by Cui et al. further reveal that MafB controls NLRP3 inflammasome activation in macrophages by maintaining p62 expression [30]. These discoveries highlight the intricate relationship between autophagy-associated proteins and inflammasome regulation, which is central to the development of chronic inflammatory diseases.

3.2 Cancer: Tumor-associated macrophages (TAMs) and immunosuppression

Tumor-associated macrophages (TAMs) are the integral components of the tumor microenvironment, and their activities are intricately modulated by autophagy [31]. Dysregulation of autophagy within TAMs can foster tumor progression *via* diverse mechanisms, with immunosuppression being a primary driver. Recent investigations have indicated that inhibiting autophagy can trigger the M2 polarization of macrophages, a process linked to a pro-tumorigenic and immunosuppressive phenotype. Gao et al. reported that in hepatocellular carcinoma, suppressed autophagy heightens the instability of the NF-κB pathway, thus promoting the M2 polarization of macrophages. M2-polarized TAMs secrete cytokines like TGF-β and IL-10, which dampen the activity of anti-tumor immune cells, including T cells and natural killer cells, enabling tumor cells to elude immune detection [32].

Autophagy also contributes significantly to the regulation of tumor metastasis by myeloid cells. Jinushi et al. demonstrated that myeloid cells regulate tumor metastasis in an autophagy-dependent manner. Tumor cells have the capacity to induce alterations in autophagy within TAMs [33]. For instance, Wang et al. discovered that tumor cells stimulate the expression of LAMP2a in TAMs, a phenomenon associated with cancer progression [34]. Moreover, Kuo et al. revealed that autophagy drives the plasticity and functional polarization of TAMs, further augmenting the immunosuppressive nature of the tumor microenvironment [35]. The interaction between autophagy and myeloid-derived suppressor cells (MDSCs) is equally crucial in the context of cancer [36]. When autophagy malfunctions in these cells, normal immune-regulatory functions are disrupted, facilitating tumor growth and metastasis.

3.3 Neurodegeneration: Defective clearance of protein aggregates

Neurodegenerative disorders, notably Alzheimer's disease (AD) and Parkinson's disease (PD), are typified by the aggregation of abnormal proteins within neurons, and autophagy is fundamental to their elimination. A defining pathological feature of AD is the buildup of amyloid-β (Aβ) plaques. Pickford et al. [37] found that beclin 1, a protein essential for autophagy, exhibits diminished expression in the early stages of AD. In mouse models, this reduction was linked to elevated Aβ accumulation. With beclin 1-dependent autophagy impaired, the removal of Aβ is compromised, triggering aggregation and subsequent neurotoxic consequences [37]. In PD, the aggregation of α-synuclein into Lewy bodies is a hallmark. Both autophagy and mitophagy within neurons are indispensable for preserving neuronal viability in PD [38, 39]. The PINK1/PARKIN signaling pathway, which orchestrates mitophagy, frequently malfunctions in PD patients [40]. Pathway defects result in the accumulation of damaged mitochondria, which release pro-apoptotic substances and reactive oxygen species (ROS), intensifying neuronal injury. Moreover, the failure of autophagy to efficiently clear α-synuclein contributes to disease progression. Li et al. demonstrated that in PD, the macrophage migration inhibitory factor exerts neuroprotective effects by modulating inflammation, apoptosis, and autophagy, underscoring the therapeutic importance of autophagy regulation [41]. Collectively, the impaired autophagic clearance of protein aggregates in neurodegenerative diseases precipitates the gradual deterioration of neuronal function and cell death, highlighting the pivotal role of autophagy in maintaining neuronal balance.

Understanding the mechanisms underlying autophagy dysregulation in these diseases provides a foundation for developing targeted therapeutic strategies. Future research should focus on exploring novel ways to modulate autophagy, either by enhancing autophagic function in neurodegenerative diseases or by inhibiting autophagy-related processes in cancer and chronic inflammation, to improve the disease management and patient outcomes.

4. Diagnostic and therapeutic implications of autophagy in macrophages

4.1 Diagnostic aspects: Biomarker panels for disease staging

Autophagy in macrophages has emerged as a critical process influencing disease progression, making it a potential source of biomarkers for clinical staging. Recent studies highlight that autophagic flux markers, such as LC3-II accumulation, p62/SQSTM1 degradation, and lysosomal activity, correlate with macrophage functional states in inflammatory and infectious diseases. For instance, in sepsis, dysregulated macrophage autophagy is linked to excessive inflammation and organ damage, suggesting that autophagic markers could stratify disease severity and predict outcomes [42]. Similarly, during an infection caused by the influenza A virus, autophagy collaborates with exosome secretion to promote the polarization of macrophages toward the M1 phenotype; exosomal cargo (e.g., miRNAs, DAMPs) may serve as non-invasive biomarkers to monitor immune activation and tissue injury [43]. Advances in multi-omics approaches further support the integration of autophagy-related proteins, miRNAs (e.g., miR-33, which regulates mitochondrial autophagy in lung fibrosis), and exosomal signatures into diagnostic panels for conditions like acute kidney injury and neurodegenerative disorders [44, 45]. Such panels could enhance precision in tracking macrophage-mediated pathophysiology across diseases.

4.2 Therapeutic aspects: Targeting autophagy in macrophages

Modulating macrophage autophagy offers promising therapeutic avenues. In infectious diseases, enhancing autophagy restricts intracellular pathogens like *Mycobacterium tuberculosis* by promoting lysosomal degradation, suggesting that mTOR inhibitors (e.g., rapamycin) or TFEB activators could bolster host defense [46]. Conversely, in hyperinflammatory states such as sepsis, fine-tuning autophagy may mitigate organ damage—pharmacological inhibitors of excessive autophagy (e.g., chloroquine) have shown potential in preclinical models [42]. In fibrotic diseases, targeting autophagy in macrophages shows organ-specific benefits. For instance, miR-33 deficiency enhances mitophagy, resolves mitochondrial stress, and attenuates lung fibrosis [47]. The absence of Atg5 in macrophages prevents kidney fibrosis through the disruption of the CCR6-CCL20 axis, thus revealing an innovative pathway for therapeutic strategies [48].

Additionally, exosome-based therapies, which exploit autophagic machinery to modulate the macrophage polarization, are being explored for regenerative purposes, such as kidney repair [45]. However, context-dependent roles of autophagy—protective or detrimental—demand careful therapeutic design. For instance, in the realm of oncology, blocking autophagy in tumor-associated macrophages has the potential to enhance the efficacy of chemotherapy through a synergistic effect. Conversely, activating autophagy pathways in these cells could reverse the state of immunosuppression prevalent in the tumor microenvironment. In the field of oncology, for example, blocking autophagy in tumor-associated macrophages has the potential to combine effectively with chemotherapy, while its activation might alleviate the immunosuppressive state [49]. The development of novel technologies, such as mitophagy-based reporting systems [50], allows for the instant evaluation of treatment outcomes. This advancement sets the stage for the creation of customized therapeutic approaches.

5. Future directions

Translating autophagy biomarkers into clinical practice and refining context-specific therapies will require deeper insights into macrophage heterogeneity and autophagic network dynamics. Collaborative efforts to map autophagic networks in macrophage subtypes across diseases will be essential for advancing diagnostics and targeted interventions.

Conflict of interest

The authors declare that there are no competing interests associated with this work.

Author details

Jiexing Tan[†], Changsheng He[†] and Li Gong*
Experimental Animal Center, Nanfang Hospital, Southern Medical University, Guangzhou, China

*Address all correspondence to: gongli009@126.com

† These authors contributed equally.

References

[1] Mizushima N, Komatsu M. Autophagy: Renovation of cells and tissues. Cell. 2011;**147**(4):728-741

[2] Pickrell AM, Youle RJ. The roles of PINK1, parkin, and mitochondrial fidelity in Parkinson's disease. Neuron. 2015;**85**(2):257-273

[3] Kaushik S, Cuervo AM. The coming of age of chaperone-mediated autophagy. Nature Reviews Molecular Cell Biology. 2018;**19**(6):365-381

[4] Sanjuan MA, Dillon CP, Tait SWG, Moshiach S, et al. Toll-like receptor signalling in macrophages links the autophagy pathway to phagocytosis. Nature. 2007;**450**(7173):1253-1257

[5] Saitoh T, Fujita N, Jang MH, et al. Loss of the autophagy protein Atg16L1 enhances endotoxin-induced IL-1β production. Nature. 2008;**456**(7219):264-268

[6] Liu K et al. Mitochondrial homeostasis and inflammation in health and disease. Cell Death and Differentiation. 2015;**22**(9):1379-1388

[7] O'Neill LA, Kishton RJ, Rathmell J. A guide to immunometabolism for immunologists. Nature Reviews Immunology. 2016;**16**(9):553-565

[8] Deretic V, Saitoh T, Akira S. Autophagy in infection, inflammation, and immunity. Nature Reviews Immunology. 2013;**13**(10):722-737

[9] Levine B, Mizushima N, Virgin HW. Autophagy in immunity and inflammation. Nature. 2011;**469**(7330):323-335

[10] Sliter DA, Martinez J, Hao L, et al. Parkin and PINK1 mitigate STING-induced inflammation. Nature. 2018;**561**(7722):258-262

[11] Zhong WZ, Rao ZQ, Xu J, et al. Defective mitophagy in aged macrophages promotes mitochondrial DNA cytosolic leakage to activate STING signaling during liver sterile inflammation. Aging Cell. 2022;**21**(6):e13622

[12] Picca A, Calvani R, Coelho-Junior HJ, Marzetti E. Cell death and inflammation: The role of mitochondria in health and disease. Cells. 2021;**10**(3):537-554

[13] Qiao L, Wang HF, Xiang L, et al. Deficient chaperone-mediated autophagy promotes lipid accumulation in macrophage. Journal of Cardiovascular Translational Research. 2021;**14**(4):661-669

[14] Kim JY, Kim SH, Kang H, et al. TFEB-GDF15 axis protects against obesity and insulin resistance as a lysosomal stress response. Nature Metabolism. 2021;**3**(3):410-427

[15] Nakahira K, Haspel JA, Rathinam VAK, Lee SJ, et al. Autophagy proteins regulate innate immune responses by inhibiting the release of mitochondrial DNA mediated by the NALP3 inflammasome. Nature Immunology. 2011;**12**(3):222-230

[16] Gutierrez MG, Master SS, Singh SB, et al. Autophagy is a defense mechanism inhibiting BCG and *Mycobacterium tuberculosis* survival in infected macrophages. Cell. 2004;**119**(6):753-766

[17] Birmingham CL, Smith AC, Bakowski MA, et al. Autophagy controls Salmonella infection in response to damage to the Salmonella-containing

vacuole. Journal of Biological Chemistry. 2006;**281**(16):11374-11383

[18] Lee J, Lee S-A, Son S-H, et al. Impaired mitophagy induces antimicrobial responses in macrophages infected with *Mycobacterium tuberculosis*. Cell & Bioscience. 2023;**13**(1):158

[19] Liu WZ, Li HL. COVID-19: Captures iron and generates reactive oxygen species to damage the human immune system. Autoimmunity. 2021;**54**(4):213-224

[20] Rubinsztein DC, Codogno P, Levine B. Autophagy modulation as a potential therapeutic target for diverse diseases. Nature Reviews. Drug Discovery. 2012;**11**(9):709-730

[21] Liu T, Wang LQ, Liang PP, et al. USP19 suppresses inflammation and promotes M2-like macrophage polarization by manipulating NLRP3 function via autophagy. Cellular & Molecular Immunology. 2021;**18**(10):2431-2442

[22] Mills EL, Kelly B, Logan A, et al. Succinate dehydrogenase supports metabolic repurposing of mitochondria to drive inflammatory macrophages. Cell. 2016;**167**(2):457-470

[23] Luo J, Wang J, Zhang J, et al. Nrf2 deficiency exacerbated CLP-induced pulmonary injury and inflammation through autophagy- and NF-κB/PPARγ-mediated macrophage polarization. Cells. 2022;**11**(23):3927

[24] Schroder K, Tschopp J. The inflammasomes. Cell. 2010;**140**(6):821-832

[25] Martinon F, Mayor A, Tschopp J. The inflammasomes: Guardians of the body. Annual Review of Immunology. 2009;**27**:229-265

[26] Zhou R, Yazdi AS, Menu P, Tschopp J. A role for mitochondria in NLRP3 inflammasome activation. Nature. 2011;**469**(7329):221-225

[27] Youle RJ, Narendra DP. Mechanisms of mitophagy. Nature Reviews. Molecular Cell Biology. 2011;**12**(1):9-14

[28] Saitoh T, Fujita N, Jang MH, et al. Loss of the autophagy protein Atg16L1 enhances endotoxin-induced IL-1beta production. Nature. 2008;**456**(7219):264-268

[29] Qiao L, Ma J, Zhang ZH, et al. Deficient chaperone-mediated autophagy promotes inflammation and atherosclerosis. Circulation Research. 2021;**129**(12):1141-1157

[30] Cui HC, Banerjee S, Xie N, et al. MafB regulates NLRP3 inflammasome activation by sustaining p62 expression in macrophages. Communications Biology. 2023;**6**(1):1047

[31] Mantovani A, Biswas SK, Galdiero MR, Sica A, Locati M. Macrophage plasticity and polarization: In vivo veritas. The Journal of Clinical Investigation. 2013;**123**(6):2410-2419

[32] Gao Z, Li XG, Feng SR, et al. Autophagy suppression facilitates macrophage M2 polarization via increased instability of NF-κB pathway in hepatocellular carcinoma. International Immunopharmacology. 2023;**123**:110685

[33] Jinushi M, Morita T, Xu ZH, et al. Autophagy-dependent regulation of tumor metastasis by myeloid cells. PLoS ONE. 2017;**12**(7):e0179357

[34] Wang RB, Liu YT, Liu L, et al. Tumor cells induce LAMP2a expression in tumor-associated macrophage for cancer progression. eBioMedicine. 2019;**40**:118-134

[35] Kuo WT, Chang JM, Chen CC, et al. Autophagy drives plasticity and functional polarization of tumor-associated macrophages. IUBMB Life. 2022;**74**(4):157-169

[36] Nie J, Wang D, Li MJ, et al. The crosstalk between autophagy and myeloid-derived suppressor cell responses in cancer. Clinical & Translational Oncology. 2023;**25**(10):2832-2840

[37] Pickford F, Masliah E, Britschgi M, et al. The autophagy-related protein beclin 1 shows reduced expression in early Alzheimer disease and regulates amyloid beta accumulation in mice. The Journal of Clinical Investigation. 2008;**118**(1):219-229

[38] Lizama BN, Chu CT. Neuronal autophagy and mitophagy in Parkinson's disease. Molecular Aspects of Medicine. 2021;**82**:100972

[39] Chu CT. Mechanisms of selective autophagy and mitophagy: Implications for neurodegenerative diseases. Neurobiology of Disease. 2019;**122**:23-34

[40] Quinn PMJ, Moreira PI, Amborsio AF, et al. PINK1/PARKIN signalling in neurodegeneration and neuroinflammation. Acta Neuropathologica Communications. 2020;**8**(1):189

[41] Li SY, Zhang QX, Guo ML, et al. Macrophage migration inhibitory factor mediates neuroprotective effects by regulating inflammation, apoptosis and autophagy in Parkinson's disease. Neuroscience. 2019;**15**(416):50-62

[42] Qiu P, Liu Y, Zhang J. Review: The role and mechanisms of macrophage autophagy in Sepsis. Inflammation. 2019;**42**(1):6-19

[43] Xia C, Xu W, Ai X, Zhu Y, Geng P, Niu Y, et al. Autophagy and exosome coordinately enhance macrophage M1 polarization and recruitment in influenza a virus infection. Frontiers in Immunology. 2022;**13**:722053

[44] Zhang XY, Wang J, Zhang J, et al. Exosomes highlight future directions in the treatment of acute kidney injury. International Journal of Molecular Sciences. 2023;**24**(21):15568

[45] Mizushima N, Levine B. Autophagy in human diseases. New England Journal of Medicine. 2020;**383**(16):1564-1576

[46] Golovkine GR, Roberts AW, Morrison HM, et al. Autophagy restricts *Mycobacterium tuberculosis* during acute infection in mice. Nature Microbiology. 2023;**8**(5):819-832

[47] Ahangari F, Price NL, Malik S, et al. microRNA-33 deficiency in macrophages enhances autophagy, improves mitochondrial homeostasis, and protects against lung fibrosis. JCI Insight. 2023;**8**(4):e158100

[48] Yufeng Z, Jiexing T, Yuanzhan W, Yuhong G, Xiaoyong Z, Ziguo Y, et al. Atg5 deficiency in macrophages protects against kidney fibrosis via the CCR6-CCL20 axis. Cell Communication and Signaling: CCS. 2024;**22**(1):223

[49] Amaravadi RK, Kimmelman AC, Debnath J. Targeting autophagy in cancer: Recent advances and future directions. Cancer Discovery. 2019;**9**(9):1167-1181

[50] Katayama HK, Hama H, Nagasawa K, et al. Visualizing and modulating mitophagy for therapeutic studies of neurodegeneration. Cell. 2020;**181**(5):1176-1187

Section 5

Macrophage Signalling: The Impact of Marine Compounds

Chapter 5

Effects of Marine Compounds on Macrophage Signaling

Jennifer Mildenberger and Céline Rebours

Abstract

Macrophages are central coordinators of innate immune responses and are involved in the inflammatory aspect of many chronic disorders. Marine compounds, such as omega-3 fatty acids or bioactive algae molecules, are known for their anti-inflammatory and antioxidative effects. There is a vast potential for new natural medicines of marine origin, and knowledge on how these affect macrophages is essential for their development. Also, a better understanding of the resulting effects of dietary intake of seafood has potential in the maintenance of inflammatory and oxidative homeostasis and prevention of chronic inflammation. This chapter gives a qualitative overview of the effects of marine fatty acids, polysaccharides, polyphenols, pigments, peptides, and few other marine compounds with a focus on known modes of action of antioxidative and immunomodulatory effects in macrophages. The relevance of these effects is also discussed in the context of chronic inflammatory diseases, which are important health challenges of our time and in which macrophages are interesting targets for modification by marine compounds.

Keywords: omega-3 fatty acids, specialized pro-resolving mediators, algae, polysaccharides, polyphenols, pigments, marine peptides

1. Introduction

Acute inflammation is crucial for the defense against pathogens, but tight regulation of inflammatory processes is essential for tissue homeostasis. Macrophages exert important functions in the acute phase of inflammation but are also initiators of resolution and repair to restore tissue homeostasis. Macrophages have a high plasticity, and their activation state is often connected to a rather pro-inflammatory (M1-like) or pro-resolving and anti-inflammatory (M2-like) polarization, while also numerous intermediate polarizations exist [1]. When inflammatory signaling becomes aberrant, chronic inflammation contributes to most non-communicated and immune-mediated inflammatory diseases (NCDs and IMIDs).

Numerous compounds from marine sources have been largely evaluated for their effects on oxidative stress and inflammatory signaling, which are tightly connected to macrophage responses as central regulators of inflammation. Most often, antioxidative effects and dampened or induced cytokine secretions are reported in this context. Marine compounds extracted from different organisms belong generally to macromolecule types such as fatty acids, polysaccharides, polyphenols, and proteins. Omega-3 polyunsaturated fatty acids (n-3 PUFAs) are best known as bioactive marine fatty acids from fish oils. However, n-3 PUFAs are initially and primarily synthesized by marine microorganisms, and then accumulate through the food chain [2]. As most molecules discussed here, n-3 PUFAs cannot be synthesized by the human body but are essential fatty acids to be taken up by diet. Marine polysaccharides are mainly found and extracted from the cell walls of macroalgae, marine microorganisms, and invertebrates, where they often have energy storage and structural functions [3]. Compared to terrestrial polysaccharides, those from marine organisms contain more sulfate groups [4], what might be correlated with their bioactivity [5, 6]. Polyphenols are naturally occurring phenols synthesized as secondary metabolites of plants for their protection against pathogens and environmental stresses. In the ocean, polyphenols are mainly found in marine algae and are more diverse and variable than polyphenols from terrestrial sources [7]. The best studied bioactive marine pigments are the carotenoids fucoxanthin and astaxanthin. Fucoxanthin is found in brown macroalgae, and astaxanthin is mainly found in microalgae and crustaceans. However, all autotrophic marine organisms such as archaea, bacteria, and yeast produce carotenoids [8]. Algae produce many of these molecules, and their bioactivities have recently been reviewed by Cadar *et al.*, providing an extensive list of compounds and their functional effects [9]. Finally, bioactive peptides obtained by hydrolysis of marine organisms have recently gained much attention for their health-beneficial effects [10]. On the other hand, antimicrobial peptides (AMP) are secondary metabolites isolated from marine sources with interest in their antimicrobial properties [11].

Overall, many reports and reviews have described the bioactive functions of these compounds from various marine sources, whereas how they modify inflammatory signaling is often less clear. This chapter presents a selection of marine compounds with examples on known modes of action in macrophages.

2. Effects of marine fatty acids

It is well established that n-3 PUFAs from marine sources have anti-inflammatory effects, and their modes of action are among the best described for marine ingredients [12, 13]. PUFAs are defined by the location of their double bounds in the carbon backbone, further giving rise to their molecular structure. It has long been known that n-6 PUFAs in cell membranes serve as substrates for the production of pro-inflammatory eicosanoids, while counteracted by n-3 PUFAs [12]. The increased incorporation of n-3 PUFAs in cell membranes was further shown to modulate lipid rafts, which are cholesterol-rich microdomains important for cellular signaling [14–16]. With regard to macrophage functions, altered lipid rafts by incorporation of the n-3 PUFA docosahexaenoic acid (DHA, 22:6 (n-3)) reduced monocyte adhesion [17] and antigen-presentation by interference with major histocompatibility complex (MHC) receptor organization [18]. Changes in lipid rafts also affect lipopolysaccharide (LPS)-induced inflammatory signaling [19]. Moreover, saturated fatty acids are needed for dimerization of toll-like receptor 4 (TLR4) and TLR2, while n-3 PUFAs inhibit this mechanism [20]. In 2010, the free fatty acid receptor 4 (FFA4/GPR120) was shown to bind n-3 PUFAs, leading to the recruitment of β-arrestin-2 that inhibits nuclear factor kappa beta (NF-κB) and Jun N-terminal kinase (JNK) pathways by sequestering the common signaling molecule TGF-beta-activated kinase 1 (TAB1) [21]. The n-3 PUFA

DHA and herring roe oil also limited interferon regulatory factor (IRF) signaling [22, 23]. Further, the intracellular receptor and transcription factor peroxisome proliferator-activated receptor gamma (PPARγ) is activated by n-3 PUFAs and involved in the polarization towards anti-inflammatory M2-like macrophages [24]. M2-like polarization was also induced by DHA-through promotion of autophagy and activation of the p38 mitogen-activated protein kinase (MAPK) [25]. N-3 PUFAs have further been reported to activate the nutrient sensor 5' AMP-activated protein kinase (AMPK), exerting an anti-inflammatory effect via sirtuin 1 (SIRT) that is deacetylating the NF-κB subunit p65 [26]. Moreover, it has been shown in rats that n-3 PUFA diet can have an impact on microRNAs in PBMCs by downregulating miR-19b-3p and miR-146b-5p [27]. We and others have shown that n-3 PUFAs activate nuclear factor (erythroid-derived 2)-like 2 (NFE2L2), an important transcription factor of the anti-oxidant response [22, 28]. We suggest a temporary increase in reactive oxygen species (ROS) and subsequent sequestration of kelch-like ECH-associated protein 1 (KEAP1) as the mechanism of NFE2L2 activation in macrophages [22]. An anti-inflammatory function of NFE2L2 signaling is well known [29]. Interestingly, monounsaturated a fatty acid from cyanobacteria has also been reported to reduce inflammatory signaling via activation of NFE2L2 [30]. On the other hand, it was proposed that DHA impairs macrophage responses towards mycobacterium tuberculosis by interfering with signal transducer and activator of transcription 1 (STAT1) phosphorylation and the localization of interferon gamma receptor in lipid rafts [31]. Overall, it seems that n-3 PUFAs are beneficial in case of infections with extracellular pathogens due to lower inflammation, while detrimental with intracellular pathogens [32].

Despite extensive mechanistical data behind the inflammation limiting effects of n-3 PUFAs in macrophages, also inconsistencies exist in clinical trials [33, 34]. This might be partly explained by the discovery that immune and other cells metabolize PUFAs to specific lipid mediators (LM), which actively promote the resolution-phase of inflammation, as described by an extensive body of work during the last decades [35–37], concisely summarized by Chiang and Serhan [38]. While n-6 PUFAs are the precursors for pro-inflammatory eicosanoids such as the leukotriene LTB_4 and the prostaglandins PGE_2 and PGF_{2a}, which play a role in the acute phase of inflammation, n-3 PUFAs can be metabolized to specialized pro-resolving mediators (SPMs) promoting resolution and repair [39]. At the peak of inflammation, central enzymes in the production of LMs (lipoxygenases (5-, 12-, and 15-LOX), cyclo-oxygenase-2 (COX2), and cytochrome P450) switch their substrate utilization from the biosynthesis of pro-inflammatory lipid mediators to the production of SPMs. Evidence exists that this switch might partly depend on the subcellular localization of the enzymes [40]. The n-3 PUFA eicosapentaenoic acid (EPA, 20:5 (n-3)) is converted to 18-HEPE and further to E-series resolvins (RvE). The metabolism of DHA leads to the formation of intermediate metabolites like 17-HDHA, 17S-hydroperoxy-DHA, and 14S-Hydroperoxy-DHA and further to respectively, D-series resolvins (RvD), protectins (PD), and maresins (MaR). The n-6 PUFA arachidonic acid (AA) also gives rise to pro-resolving lipoxins (LXA_4 and LXB_4). More recently, the synthesis of docosapentaenoic acid (DPA, 22:5 (n-3))-derived RvDs, PDs, and MaRs has been described [41, 42] as well as cysteinyl-conjugated SPMs-termed conjugates in tissue regeneration (CTR) [43]. The activity of SPMs is mediated through binding to their respective G-protein coupled receptors (GPCR/GPR) like the formylpeptide receptor 2 (FPR2/ALX), the RvD1 and LXA_4 receptor GPR32, chemokine-like receptor 1 (CMKLR1/ChemR23), the LTB_4 receptor (LBT4R/BLT1), and GPR18 [44]. Macrophages are central cells in the production of and response to all types of SPMs [38, 39] and are the main source of MaRs and their CTR (MCTR) [45]. Interestingly, while pro-resolving LM synthesis was first described in polymorphonuclear cells (PMN), it was also shown that microparticles from PMNs as well as phagocytosis of apoptotic PMNs (efferocytosis) provide substrates and promote LM synthesis in macrophages [46]. Overall, the different classes of SPMs share pro-resolving effects on macrophages, such as increased efferocytosis, reduced inflammatory signaling, and promotion of a pro-resolution polarization [39]. The induction of phagocytosis/efferocytosis in macrophages is a hallmark of SPM-mediated effects and directly linked to active resolving and repair [47]. Interestingly, the receptor ChemR23 is only expressed in M1 type macrophages. ChemR23 is the receptor for chemerin, which is attracting monocytes/macrophages to the site of insult. The initiation of resolution further leads to repolarization of these macrophages to a pro-resolution type by the binding of RvE1 to Chem23 [48]. It has been shown that the LM profile produced by macrophages depends on the macrophage lineage and type of stimuli [40, 49]. Importantly, the supplementation of human macrophages with different marine fish- or algae-derived oils promoted the synthesis of distinct LM profiles [50, 51]. Moreover, LM-enriched oils promoted resolving-associated macrophage and microglia phenotypes in man and mice [52, 53]. It is well established that SPMs exert their effects via binding to GPCRs leading to various pro-resolving downstream effects that might also overlap with or explain mechanisms described for n-3 PUFAs. Especially the fact that different SPMs bind to several GPCRs, and multiple SPMs bind to each receptor leads to complex pathways between receptors and effects, with details reviewed elsewhere [47, 54]. To mention some mechanisms, the activation of the six described SPM-binding GPCRs often involves the recruitment of β-arrestin, mediating further effects via among others modulation of calcium release, cyclic adenosine monophosphate (cAMP) signaling, and on transcription factor activity of NF-κB, MAPKs, and STAT3 [54]. Furthermore, regulation of microRNAs has been described as part of SPM effects [55]. The SPM-induced increase in phagocytosis is also explained by GPCR activation leading to cytoskeletal changes [56, 57].

Finally, although most research has been done in mammals, the synthesis of SPMs takes place throughout the food chain and SPMs as well as their precursors can be found in microalgae and fish [58, 59].

3. Effects of marine polysaccharides

Many types of marine polysaccharides are reported to have anti-inflammatory or immunostimulatory effects as well as to modulate ROS signaling by their antioxidative capacities. The sulfate content in marine polysaccharides was suggested to be correlated with their radical scavenging activity [5, 6]. Sulfated polysaccharides, extracted from brown macroalgae, have been reported to reduce cytokine secretions as well as to limit the activity of NF-κB and MAPKs in macrophages [60], and also immune-stimulating effects have been reported [61]; also, we have shown that both effects might co-exist, depending on the basal inflammatory status [62]. Observations in porcine monocytes and alveolar macrophages support the induction of an immune tolerance state by the treatment with sulphated polysaccharides [63], whereas we have shown that polysaccharide-rich macroalgae extracts specifically downregulated IRF-signaling [62]. Alginate oligosaccharides were shown to bind TLR4 to activate pro-inflammatory signaling [64], while much research is ongoing to optimize pro-resolving and tissue restoring effects of alginate hydrogels in biomedical applications

[65]. Although less studied, ulvan from green macroalgae was also reported with both anti-inflammatory and immunomodulatory function [66]. Ascophyllan, a sulphated polysaccharide from *Ascophyllum nodosum*, strongly activated the transcription factors NF-κB and AP-1 and the secretion of pro-inflammatory cytokines [67]. A sulphated polysaccharide from red macroalgae reduced LPS-induced ROS and NO signaling and NF-κB and MAPK signaling [68]. Microalgae polysaccharides inhibited the activation of MAPK/NF-κB, PI3K/AKT, and STAT-3 pathways and activated NFE2L2 signaling [69]. A bacillus proteoglycan has been shown to suppress macrophage inflammatory signaling by reduced protein levels of MAPKs and NF-κB subunit p65, possibly due to increased ubiquitination and degradation [70]. Chitooligosaccharide obtained after hydrolysis of shrimp shell chitosan reduced LPS-induced ROS and the expression of the NFE2L2 target heme oxygenase (HMOX1) as well as the phosphorylation of PKB/Akt and extracellular-signal regulated kinases 1/2 (ERK1/2) [71]. Clam polysaccharides promoted a shift from M2 to M1-like in tumor-associated macrophages (TAMs), thus increasing their anti-cancer activity [72].

As hydrophilic macromolecules, polysaccharides do not have the capability to freely cross the cell membrane but need to interact with receptors. This is well described for fucoidans, a group of marine sulphated polysaccharides found in brown macroalgae as well as the body wall of certain marine organisms such as sea cucumbers [73]. Fucoidan has long been used as ligand for the class A scavenger receptor (SR-A, CD204) in macrophages [74, 75]. SRs recognize and internalize molecules such as low-density lipoprotein (LDL), LPS, and lipoteichoic acid (LTA), and also marine polysaccharides might be internalized through receptor interactions. SR-A lacks the cytoplasmatic activation site but co-operates with other receptors such as TLR4 to mediate fucoidan effects. The binding of fucoidan to SR-A might also hinder the binding of other factors and their functions. Furthermore, TLRs, C-type lectins, selectins, and other receptors have been reported as molecular targets of fucoidan mediating their respective effects [75, 76]. Likewise, brown algae fucoidan was suggested to increase TNF-α secretion through receptor interaction [77]. It is further acknowledged that the structure of fucoidans is an important factor for their biological activity and Apostolova *et al.* give an overview on the effects of algae-derived fucoidans [61].

Chen et al. have shown that the inhibitory effect of fucoidan on the NLRP3 inflammasome in oxidized LDL (oxLDL) macrophages, a model for foam cells, depends on the ability of fucoidan to up-regulate selective autophagy [78]. Also, sea cucumber fucoidan was able to upregulate autophagy to limit the expression of cytokines and inflammasome components [79]. The relation of autophagy and the inflammasome is well described as inflammasome components are targeted to selective autophagy, namely, recognized by selective autophagy receptors, which link them to the autophagy machinery, being engulfed in autophagosomes and finally recycled by fusion with lysosomes [80]. How exactly fucoidans and possibly other marine polysaccharides induce autophagy is not described; however, a connection between TLR activation and autophagy exists [81]. On the other hand, it has also been proposed that fucoidan inhibits autophagy in endoplasmatic reticulum (ER)-stressed macrophages via activation of SR-A and mechanistic target of rapamycin (mTOR) [82]. Thus, fucoidan effects might differ depending on other active cellular signaling. Fucoidan was also able to reduce lipid accumulation and increase the efflux of cholesterol from induced oxLDL macrophages by increased expression of ATP-binding cassette transporter A1 (ABCA1) possibly via liver X receptor-α (LXR-α) [83]. In another study, fucoidan reduced the production of colony stimulating factor 1 (CSF1) and thereby limited migration and cytokine production of macrophages [84]. Importantly, polysaccharides might undergo modifications during digestion, and in this regard it was shown that fucoidan after simulated fecal fermentation induced nitric oxide (NO) production, cytokine secretion and phagocytosis [85].

In the light of diverse possible receptor interactions, recurrent patterns are present, but specific effects of polysaccharides seem to depend on the exact molecules present, timing, and cellular state. This might need to be tested rather than deduced.

4. Effects of marine polyphenols

Polyphenols are a large group of reactive molecules and are best known for their ROS scavenging effects [86]. Detailed classification and structures of marine polyphenols are found elsewhere [87]. Phlorotannins are a group of polyphenols that are abundant in certain brown macroalgae, and their antioxidative and anti-inflammatory effects have been reviewed [88]. Many phlorotannins have been shown to reduce ROS and NF-κB activity. Likewise, phlorotannins from *Fucus vesiculosus* blocked NF-κB activation by inhibiting the phosphorylation and degradation of NF-kappa-B inhibitor alpha (IκB) [89]. Also, two bieckols, phlorotannins from *Ecklonia cava*, supressed NF-κB activity, possibly partly through limiting LPS-induced ROS [90, 91] and a dieckol reduced fine-dust-induced ROS via increased superoxide dismutase production as well as activation of NFE2L2 [92]. Similarly, fucofuroeckol-A from *Eisenia bicyclis* reduced NF-κB and MAPK activation [93]. Interestingly, an eckol from *E. cava* activated NFE2L2 through activation of ERK and PKB/Akt [94]. Inhibitory effects of phlorotannins have been demonstrated on secretory phospholipase A_2s ($sPLA_2$s), LOXs and COXs, all of which are involved in the metabolism of the endogenous n-6 PUFA arachidonic acid (AA) to pro-inflammatory prostaglandins [95, 96]. Flavonoids from macroalgae are far less studied, but a polyhydroxyflavone extracted from the brown seaweed *Hizikia fusiforme* was shown to limit NF-κB activation through stabilization of IκB-α [97]. Many of the phenolic compounds (such as catechin, quercetin, kaempferol) are mainly studied from terrestrial plants; however, as they are also found in marine micro- and macroalgae, similar effects would be expected. In this regard, the flavonoid kaempferol inhibited NF-κB and MAPK signaling and limited macrophage M1-like polarization [98]. Quercetin reduced ROS formation and thus activation of the inflammasome, as well as limited TLR2 expression and AMPK phosphorylation, activated NFE2L2 and promoted M2-like polarization [99]. As an example of other phenolics, bromophenols from red macroalgae dampened inflammatory signaling by reducing LPS-induced ROS and ERK1/2 phosphorylation [100] and reduced NF-κB and STAT1 phosphorylation [101].

Taken together, marine polyphenols might limit ROS, activate antioxidative and detoxifying enzymes, and inhibit central inflammatory transcription factors. Interestingly, polyphenols were also reported to interfere with lipid rafts, what could at least partly explain their anti-inflammatory effects [102].

5. Effects of marine pigments

Carotenoids from marine sources and their health-related effects have been recently reviewed [8], while we focus here on the most commonly described pigments. Fucoxanthin is a xanthophyll carotenoid found in brown algae with antioxidant and anti-inflammatory effects [103]. It has been shown that fucoxanthin is able to upregulate NFE2L2 with cytoprotective, antioxidative, and anti-inflammatory downstream effects [104–107]. The induction of NFE2L2 by fucoxanthin has been proposed to be partly mediated through direct interaction with KEAP1, the negative regulator of NFE2L2, leading to the liberation and nuclear translocation of NFE2L2 [108]. Also, interactions of fucoxanthin with upstream kinases Fyn (p59-FYN), glycogen synthase kinase-3 beta (GSK-3β), and PKB/Akt were modeled, explaining the activation of NFE2L2 [106]. Furthermore, fucoxanthin increased the expression of SIRT1 [105]. SIRT1 is a protein deacetylase involved in the regulation of several cell protective pathways such as the antioxidative response, energy maintenance, apoptosis, and senescence and has been proposed to activate NFE2L2 by its deacetylation function [109]. Fucoxanthin from the microalgae *Phaeodactylum tricornutum* was shown to limit the assembly and activation of the NLRP3 inflammasome as well as the NF-κB-dependent priming step in bone marrow-derived macrophages [110]. During digestion, fucoxanthin is hydrolysed to fucoxanthinol, which has been shown to inhibit the lysosomal enzyme N-acylethanolamine acid amidase (NAAA) and thus prevent the cleavage of the endogenous and anti-inflammatory LM palmitoylethanolamide [111]. Carotenoids from marine bacteria have also been shown to reduce NO production, TNF-α secretion, and lipid peroxidation in LPS-stimulated PBMCs [112], suggesting an inhibitory effect on NF-κB, which is however also found for other carotenoids than from marine sources [113]. Microalgae produce chlorophylls that are needed for photosynthesis as well as carotenoids and phycobiliproteins as accessory pigments, which also scavenge ROS and limit NF-κB signaling [114, 115].

Astaxanthin is a red carotenoid found mainly in microalgae and the shell of crustaceans. Mechanisms of an anti-inflammatory effect of astaxanthin have been recently summarized and include inhibition of NF-κB, MAPKs and STAT3 as well as ROS and activation of PI3K and NFE2L2 [116]. In microglia, an anti-inflammatory effect by astaxanthin was explained by the downregulation of miR-31-5p [117]. Astaxanthin has also been reported to induce NFE2L2 via increased expression of SIRT1 [118]. The activation of NFE2L2 by astaxanthin has further been linked to the prevention of macrophage ferroptosis and thus alleviating arthrosclerosis [119] and astaxanthin activated PI3K and CDC42 to increase lipid efflux from macrophages preventing the emergence of foam cells [120]. The latter was also demonstrated to depend on an increased expression of circular RNA tripeptidyl-peptidase II (circTPP2), leading to downregulation of miR-3073b-5p and upregulation of ABCA1 [121]. Astaxanthin was further suggested to cell-specifically activate PPARγ in macrophages, increasing the expression of LXR, CD36 and ABCA1 to promote lipid efflux and to mediate an anti-inflammatory effect [122].

Finally, and as an interesting fact, melanin nanoparticles from cuttlefish ink have been proposed to limit ROS and modulate macrophage polarization towards M2 [123].

6. Effects of marine peptides

Antimicrobial peptides (AMPs) are part of the remarkable defense mechanism of marine invertebrates and interesting drug candidates against antibiotic-resistant bacteria [124]. Some AMPs have been further modified to improve their antibacterial functions, and many AMPs are reported to exert antibacterial effects intracellularly in macrophages. Likewise, the marine peptide-N6NH2 and its derivatives have been shown to be internalized by macrophages though lipid rafts, micropinocytosis, and microtubule polymerization and to exert intracellular antimicrobial effects against different bacterial strains [125, 126]. Also, marine peptide-N2 conjugated with cell penetrating peptides could enter macrophages through micropinocytosis and clathrin-mediated endocytosis to reduce intracellular *Salmonella typhimurium* [127]. Hepcidin-2 from mudskipper increased the bactericidal and phagocytic function of its monocytes and macrophages [128]. Hsieh *et al.* have shown that the grouper AMP Epinecidin (Epi)-1 induces several changes in the transcriptome of LPS-stimulated macrophages, such as reducing the expression of pro-inflammatory cytokines and increasing MHC-related gene expression thought to increase the host response against LPS [129]. Perthamide C, a secondary metabolite from marine sponge, was shown to modulate the expression of chaperones such as Hsp-90 in murine macrophages, what the authors link to apoptosis reduction [130].

Bioactive peptides are also obtained from the hydrolysis of marine organisms and well known for their radical scavenging and antioxidative capacities, but often, these effects are determined biochemically and not directly transferrable into cell systems. However, peptides from hydrolyzed sea cucumber collagen were able to protect RAW264.7 macrophages from H_2O_2 induced damage by reduction of ROS and lipid oxidation and activation of antioxidant enzymes [131]. Peptides from hydrolysis of oyster soft tissue and salmon bones reduced inflammatory signaling in LPS-stimulated macrophages [132, 133], similarly to blue mussel peptides, which inhibited IκB-α and MAPK phosphorylation [134]. Anti-inflammatory peptides have also been isolated from red seaweed hydrolysate, showing mainly upregulation of IL-10 via NF-κB and MAPK activation [135]. On the other hand, Lin *et al.* purified an immunostimulatory peptide from sandworm hydrolysate, which increased macrophage proliferation, phagocytosis, and cytokine secretion [136]. Two peptides from ark shell hydrolysate activated PPAR-γ/LXR-α in macrophages treated with oxLDL, thus inhibiting the formation of foam cells [137].

7. Effects of other marine compounds

There exists a variety of further secondary metabolites from marine organisms, of which some have been described for functional effects in macrophages. To mention some, macrolactins from marine microorganisms have shown anti-inflammatory effects by the activation of NFE2L2 and BTB domain and CNC homolog 1 (BACH1) [138]. The hemiterpene equisetin, which was isolated from fungus of marine sponge, inhibited inflammatory signaling in macrophages and foam cell formation by binding and inhibiting STAT3 [139]. Gliotoxin from marine fungi promoted autophagy via increased expression of microtubule-associated proteins 1A/1B light chain 3B (MAP1LC3B/LC3) and autophagy-related 5 (ATG5) and suppressed infection by mycobacteria tuberculosis in macrophages, while no change in inflammatory signaling was observed [140]. Brevenal, a bioactive dinoflagellate compound inhibited TNF-α and IL-1β from macrophages [141]. Fucosterol, a secondary metabolite of the brown algae *Padina boryana* protected macrophages from particulate matter induced stress by reducing ROS as well as NF-κB and MAPK expression or phosphorylation [142]. Moreover, Trabectedin, a tunicate-derived alkaloid and anti-cancer drug induces caspase-8-mediated apoptosis specifically in macrophages and thus also TAMs, thereby limiting their pro-cancer effects [143].

Vitamins are essential organic micronutrients and seaweeds are rich in vitamin B-complex (folic acid and B12), vitamin C and vitamin A precursor β-carotene

[144]. Furthermore, tocopherols (Vitamin E) are produced by algae as secondary metabolites and known for their antioxidant and anti-inflammatory effects, mostly described from terrestrial plants [145–147]. Vitamin D has been produced by plankton for millions of years and has become an important hormone regulating calcium homeostasis in more complex organisms [148]. Fish is a dietary source for vitamin D. Interestingly, macrophages can both produce and respond to the active vitamin D metabolite 1,25-dihydroxyvitamin D_3 (1,25D). The multiple immunoregulatory effects of Vitamin D are described elsewhere [149].

8. Discussion

This review presents many examples on the regulation of macrophage function by marine compounds. Although the described compounds are highly diverse molecules, several recurrent pathway modifications can be delineated and include limited ROS signaling, activation of the antioxidative defense system via NFE2L2 and limited or induced activity of the main inflammatory transcription factors such as NF-κB, MAPKs and STATs, and their upstream signaling proteins. An overview of these effects is summarized in **Table 1**.

As important mode of action, n-3 PUFAs and polyphenols might incorporate into and modulate cell membranes and lipid rafts and thereby interfere with receptor signaling. N-3 PUFAs as well as their metabolites can further directly bind their specific receptors, while polysaccharides might bind to and function as agonist or

	N-3 PUFAs and metabolites	**Polysaccharides**	**Polyphenols**	**Pigments (carotenoids)**	**Peptides**
Modulation of cell membranes and lipid rafts	Inflamm. ↓		Inflamm. ↓		
Signaling via specific receptors	Inflamm. ↓				
Modulation of PRR signaling		Inflamm. ↕			
ROS scavengers/ inducers	ROS ↑ (mildly)	ROS ↓	ROS ↓	ROS ↓	ROS ↓
Modulation of intracellular proteins		Inflamm. ↕	Inflamm. ↕	Inflamm. ↕	Inflamm. ↓
Altering microRNAs	Inflamm. ↓			Inflamm. ↓	
Induction of efferocytosis	Inflamm. ↓ (Repair ↑)				
Autophagy activation	Inflamm. ↓	Inflamm. ↓			
NFE2L2 activation	ROS ↓ Inflamm. ↓		ROS ↓ Inflamm. ↓	ROS ↓ Inflamm. ↓	ROS ↓ Inflamm. ↓

Table 1.
Brief overview on reported mechanisms of marine compounds affecting macrophages and resulting in up (↑) or down (↓) modulation of inflammatory and ROS signaling.

antagonist of several pattern recognition receptors (PRR). Polysaccharides, polyphenols, and carotenoids are able to scavenge ROS by their molecular structure and might also directly interact with different enzymes and signaling proteins to modify their activity. Interestingly, polyphenols were reported to modulate the activity of lipid-metabolizing enzymes [95, 96]. Thus, there could be a potential of marine compounds other than fatty acids to modulate the resolution phase of inflammation by targeting the involved enzymes, what should be further explored.

Macrophage signaling is tightly connected to the regulation of inflammatory processes. Acute inflammation is essential in the defense from pathogens; however, when resolving mechanisms fail, macrophage signaling becomes detrimental, maintaining chronic inflammation and leading to tissue damage [150]. Chronic low-grade inflammation has been recognized as a common characteristic and underlying cause of NCDs and IMIDs [151]. The causes of chronic inflammation are many but often involve an overproduction of ROS [152]. Thus, scavenging of ROS or the activation of the antioxidative response by marine compounds counteracts this driver of chronic inflammation. Marine compounds might further modulate the subsequently and inappropriately activated inflammatory signaling pathways, which also promote the progression of associated diseases [153]. Of note, several marine compounds were reported to interfere with lipid handling in macrophages and foam cell development, playing a role in atherosclerosis. Compared to immunosuppressive drugs, which also compromise inflammatory processes that are needed in the defense from pathogens, natural compounds from the ocean might be used in prevention and milder disease to modulate macrophage functions and restore homeostasis. Especially the fact that marine compounds have often many targets suggests their use as holistic approach to limit chronic inflammation. Further, many marine organisms (and especially algae) contain an array of the above described molecules, and thus dietary intake of seafood has the potential to maintain and restore macrophage function. It is however challenging to fully understand dietary applications, where synergistic or antagonistic effects by the contained compounds might occur [153]. Moreover, polysaccharides, polyphenols, and peptides among others might be metabolized during digestion. Thus, it should be kept in mind that *in vitro* experiments do not necessarily always reflect what metabolites could be available in the blood after dietary intake of marine compounds, and further research is needed to better elucidate this aspect.

As we focus on signaling in macrophages, many of the included studies were done *in vitro* and we have not made a difference depending on what types of macrophages (human, mouse, cell lines) were used, although this might have an influence on certain results. Finally, regulation of macrophage functions is always a two-sided sword. Likewise, even though anti-inflammatory and antioxidative effects are beneficial in the treatment of IMIDs, these effects could also worsen the outcome such as reduced clearance of bacterial infections in case of too little inflammatory signaling or promotion of alternatively activated M2-like TAMs, so care has to be taken in such settings.

9. Conclusion

The ocean is a source of highly diverse bioactive compounds, and especially algae are often producers of a multitude of the here discussed compounds. Despite the diversity of compounds, certain principles in the regulation of macrophage responses are recurring, such as scavenging of ROS, activation of the antioxidative defense system, or changes in the activation of the main inflammatory transcription factors. Much research has been done on marine fatty acids, revealing their metabolism to pro-resolving LMs and SPMs. Macrophages are central in the production and response to SPMs and actively contribute to the resolution of inflammation by increased phagocytosis, a hallmark of SPM action. Algae-derived polysaccharides, polyphenols, tocopherols, and pigments are also increasingly described. While their effects are relevant for many cell types, antioxidative and immunomodulating effects have an important impact on macrophage signaling with relevance for inflammatory conditions. Finally, marine compounds often have pleiotropic effects on multiple pathways in inflammation and oxidative stress, what makes them especially interesting for the prevention and treatment of chronic inflammatory diseases.

Acknowledgements

The writing of this chapter was supported by the Norwegian Research Council (nos. 342654, 319577, and 326803), the COST Action (no. 20106), and Møreforsking AS. Jesmond Dalli is acknowledged for his valuable comments on the manuscript.

Conflict of interest

The authors declare no conflict of interest.

Author details

Jennifer Mildenberger* and Céline Rebours
Møreforsking AS, Borgundveien, Ålesund, Norway

*Address all correspondence to: jennifer.mildenberger@moreforsking.no

References

[1] Li C, Xu MM, Wang K, et al. Macrophage polarization and metainflammation. Translational Research. 2017;**191**:29

[2] Biotechnology B, Tian L, Chi G, et al. Marine microorganisms: Natural factories for polyunsaturated fatty acid production. Blue Biotechnology. 2024;**1**:1-13

[3] Carrasqueira J, Bernardino S, Bernardino R, et al. Marine-derived polysaccharides and their potential health benefits in nutraceutical applications. Marine Drugs. 2025;**23**:60

[4] Guan X, Wang F, Zhou B, et al. The nutritional function of active polysaccharides from marine animals: A review. Food Bioscience. 2024;**58**:103693

[5] Qi H, Zhang Q, Zhao T, et al. Antioxidant activity of different sulfate content derivatives of polysaccharide extracted from Ulva pertusa (Chlorophyta) in vitro. International Journal of Biological Macromolecules. 2005;**37**:195-199

[6] Wang J, Zhang Q, Zhang Z, et al. Potential antioxidant and anticoagulant capacity of low molecular weight fucoidan fractions extracted from Laminaria japonica. International Journal of Biological Macromolecules. 2010;**46**:6-12

[7] Mateos R, Pérez-Correa JR, Domínguez H. Bioactive properties of marine phenolics. Marine Drugs. 2020;**18**:501

[8] Mapelli-Brahm P, Gómez-Villegas P, Gonda ML, et al. Microalgae, seaweeds and aquatic bacteria, archaea, and yeasts: Sources of carotenoids with potential antioxidant and anti-inflammatory health-promoting actions in the sustainability era. Marine Drugs. 2023;**21**:340

[9] Cadar E, Popescu A, Dragan AML, et al. Bioactive compounds of marine algae and their potential health and nutraceutical applications: A review. Marine Drugs. 2025;**23**:152

[10] Wang P, Zhang Y, Hu J, et al. Bioactive peptides from marine organisms. Protein and Peptide Letters. 2024;**31**:569-585

[11] Wang S, Fan L, Pan H, et al. Antimicrobial peptides from marine animals: Sources, structures, mechanisms and the potential for drug development. Frontiers in Marine Science. 2023;**9**:1112595

[12] Calder PC. Marine omega-3 fatty acids and inflammatory processes: Effects, mechanisms and clinical relevance. Biochimica et Biophysica Acta - Molecular and Cell Biology of Lipids. 2015;**1851**:469-484

[13] Grytten E, Laupsa-Borge J, Cetin K, et al. Inflammatory markers after supplementation with marine n-3 or plant n-6 PUFAs: A randomized double-blind crossover study. Journal of Lipid Research. 2025;**66**:100770

[14] Pike LJ. Rafts defined: A report on the keystone symposium on lipid rafts and cell function. Journal of Lipid Research. 2006;**47**:1597-1598

[15] Wassall SR, Brzustowicz MR, Shaikh SR, et al. Order from disorder, corralling cholesterol with chaotic lipids: The role of polyunsaturated lipids in membrane raft formation. Chemistry and Physics of Lipids. 2004;**132**:79-88

[16] Hellwing C, Tigistu-Sahle F, Fuhrmann H, et al. Lipid composition of membrane microdomains isolated detergent-free from PUFA supplemented RAW264.7 macrophages. Journal of Cellular Physiology. 2018;**233**:2602-2612

[17] Schaefer MB, Schaefer CA, Schifferings S, et al. N-3 vs. n-6 fatty acids differentially influence calcium signalling and adhesion of inflammatory activated monocytes: Impact of lipid rafts. Inflammation Research. 2016;**65**:881-894

[18] Rockett BD, Carraway K, Shaikh SR. N-3 polyunsaturated fatty acid incorporates directly into lipid rafts to disrupt domain clustering and MHC lateral organization of antigen presenting cells. Biophysical Journal. 2010;**98**:425a

[19] Koseki M, Hirano KI, Masuda D, et al. Increased lipid rafts and accelerated lipopolysaccharide-induced tumor necrosis factor-α secretion in Abca1-deficient macrophages. Journal of Lipid Research. 2007;**48**:299-306

[20] Hwang DH, Kim JA, Lee JY. Mechanisms for the activation of toll-like receptor 2/4 by saturated fatty acids and inhibition by docosahexaenoic acid. European Journal of Pharmacology. 2016;**785**:24

[21] Oh DY, Talukdar S, Bae EJ, et al. GPR120 is an omega-3 fatty acid receptor mediating potent anti-inflammatory and insulin-sensitizing effects. Cell. 2010;**142**:687-698

[22] Mildenberger J, Johansson I, Sergin I, et al. N-3 PUFAs induce inflammatory tolerance by formation of KEAP1-containing SQSTM1/p62-bodies and activation of NFE2L2. Autophagy. 2017;**13**:1664-1678

[23] Mildenberger J, Solberg NT, Østbye T-KK, et al. Herring roe oil exerts anti-psoriatic and immunomodulatory effects on the IL-17/23 signaling axis in macrophages, T-cells and a keratinocyte and fibroblast co-culture. bioRxiv. 2025;**04**(22):650092

[24] Chang HY, Lee HN, Kim W, et al. Docosahexaenoic acid induces M2 macrophage polarization through peroxisome proliferator-activated receptor γ activation. Life Sciences. 2015;**120**:39-47

[25] Kawano A, Ariyoshi W, Yoshioka Y, et al. Docosahexaenoic acid enhances M2 macrophage polarization via the p38 signaling pathway and autophagy. Journal of Cellular Biochemistry. 2019;**120**:12604-12617

[26] Xue B, Yang Z, Wang X, et al. Omega-3 polyunsaturated fatty acids antagonize macrophage inflammation via activation of AMPK/SIRT1 pathway. PLoS One. 2012;**7**:e45990

[27] Zheng Z, Ge Y, Zhang J, et al. PUFA diets alter the microRNA expression profiles in an inflammation rat model. Molecular Medicine Reports. 2015;**11**:4149

[28] Davinelli S, Medoro A, Intrieri M, et al. Targeting NRF2–KEAP1 axis by Omega-3 fatty acids and their derivatives: Emerging opportunities against aging and diseases. Free Radical Biology and Medicine. 2022;**193**:736-750

[29] Saha S, Buttari B, Panieri E, et al. An overview of Nrf2 signaling pathway and its role in inflammation. Molecules. 2020;**25**:5474

[30] Al-Awadhi FH, Simon EF, Liu N, et al. Discovery and anti-inflammatory activity of a cyanobacterial fatty acid

targeting the Keap1/Nrf2 pathway. Marine Drugs. 2023;**21**:553

[31] Bonilla DL, Ly LH, Fan Y-Y, et al. Incorporation of a dietary omega 3 fatty acid impairs murine macrophage responses to mycobacterium tuberculosis. PLoS One. 2010;**5**:e10878

[32] Husson MO, Ley D, Portal C, et al. Modulation of host defence against bacterial and viral infections by omega-3 polyunsaturated fatty acids. Journal of Infection. 2016;**73**:523-535

[33] Shekarchizadeh-Esfahani P, Khaghani L, Karimian J. Effects of fish oil supplementation on serum C-reactive protein levels in trained individuals: A systematic review of clinical trials. Clinical Nutrition Research. 2025;**14**:139

[34] Li R, Wang Y, Xu J, et al. Effects of n-3 polyunsaturated fatty acid supplementation on cardiovascular indices in type 2 diabetes: A meta-analysis of randomized controlled trials. Reviews in Cardiovascular Medicine. 2025;**26**(2):25882. DOI: 10.31083/RCM25882

[35] Serhan CN. Pro-resolving lipid mediators are leads for resolution physiology. Nature. 2014;**510**:92-101

[36] Dalli J, Serhan CN. Identification and structure elucidation of the pro-resolving mediators provides novel leads for resolution pharmacology. British Journal of Pharmacology. 2019;**176**:1024-1037

[37] Serhan CN, Clish CB, Brannon J, et al. Novel functional sets of lipid-derived mediators with antiinflammatory actions generated from omega-3 fatty acids via cyclooxygenase 2–nonsteroidal antiinflammatory drugs and transcellular processing. The Journal of Experimental Medicine. 2000;**192**:1197

[38] Chiang N, Serhan CN. Specialized pro-resolving mediator network: An update on production and actions. Essays in Biochemistry. 2020;**64**:443-462

[39] Julliard WA, Myo YPA, Perelas A, et al. Specialized pro-resolving mediators as modulators of immune responses. Seminars in Immunology. 2022;**59**:101605

[40] Werz O, Gerstmeier J, Libreros S, et al. Human macrophages differentially produce specific resolvin or leukotriene signals that depend on bacterial pathogenicity. Nature Communications. 2018;**9**(1):59. DOI: 10.1038/s41467-017-02538-5

[41] Dalli J, Colas RA, Serhan CN. Novel n-3 Immunoresolvents: Structures and actions. Scientific Reports. 2013;**3**:1-15

[42] Ervik K, Reinertsen AF, Koenis DS, et al. Stereoselective synthesis, pro-resolution, and anti-inflammatory actions of RvD5n-3 DPA. Journal of Natural Products. 2023;**86**:2546-2553

[43] Serhan CN, Chiang N, Dalli J. New pro-resolving n-3 mediators bridge resolution of infectious inflammation to tissue regeneration. Molecular Aspects of Medicine. 2018;**64**:1-17

[44] Chiang N, Serhan CN. Structural elucidation and physiologic functions of specialized pro-resolving mediators and their receptors. Molecular Aspects of Medicine. 2017;**58**:114-129

[45] Dalli J, Vlasakov I, Riley IR, et al. Maresin conjugates in tissue regeneration biosynthesis enzymes in human macrophages. Proceedings of the National Academy of Sciences of the United States of America. 2016;**113**:12232-12237

[46] Dalli J, Serhan CN. Pro-resolving mediators in regulating and conferring

macrophage function. Frontiers in Immunology. 2017;**8**:1400

[47] Decker C, Sadhu S, Fredman G. Pro-resolving ligands orchestrate phagocytosis. Frontiers in Immunology. 2021;**12**:660865. DOI: 10.3389/fimmu.2021.660865

[48] Herová M, Schmid M, Gemperle C, et al. ChemR23, the receptor for Chemerin and Resolvin E1, is expressed and functional on M1 but not on M2 macrophages. The Journal of Immunology. 2015;**194**:2330-2337

[49] Radmark O. Formation of eicosanoids and other oxylipins in human macrophages. Biochemical Pharmacology. 2022;**204**:115210

[50] Sobrino A, Walker ME, Colas RA, et al. Protective activities of distinct omega-3 enriched oils are linked to their ability to upregulate specialized pro-resolving mediators. PLoS One. 2020;**15**:e0242543

[51] Ringheim-Bakka T, Saliani A, Østbye T-KK, et al. Phospholipid Esters from Herring Roe Promotes SPM Biosynthesis in Human Monocyte-Derived Macrophages and a Keratinocyte/Fibroblast co-Culture with Implications for the Treatment of Psoriasis. BioRxiv. Cold Spring Harbor; 2025

[52] Olivares-González L, Velasco S, Gallego I, et al. An SPM-enriched marine oil supplement shifted microglia polarization toward M2, ameliorating retinal degeneration in rd10 mice. Antioxidants. 2022;**12**:98

[53] Irún P, Carrera-Lasfuentes P, Sánchez-Luengo M, et al. Pharmacokinetics and changes in lipid mediator profiling after consumption of specialized pro-resolving lipid-mediator-enriched marine oil in healthy subjects. International Journal of Molecular Sciences. 2023;**24**:16143

[54] Park J, Langmead CJ, Riddy DM. New advances in targeting the resolution of inflammation: Implications for specialized pro-resolving mediator GPCR drug discovery. ACS Pharmacology and Translational Science. 2020;**3**:88

[55] Recchiuti A, Serhan CN. Pro-resolving lipid mediators (SPMs) and their actions in regulating miRNA in novel resolution circuits in inflammation. Frontiers in Immunology. 2012;**3**:298. DOI: 10.3389/fimmu.2012.00298

[56] Ohira T, Arita M, Omori K, et al. Resolvin E1 receptor activation signals phosphorylation and phagocytosis. Journal of Biological Chemistry. 2010;**285**:3451-3461

[57] Reville K, Crean JK, Vivers S, et al. Lipoxin A4 redistributes myosin IIA and Cdc42 in macrophages: Implications for phagocytosis of apoptotic leukocytes. The Journal of Immunology. 2006;**176**:1878-1888

[58] Jagusch H, Werner M, Koenis D, et al. 14,17,18-trihydroxy-eicosatetraenoic acid: A novel pro-resolving lipid mediator from marine microalgae. ACS Pharmacology and Translational Science. 2021;**4**:1188-1194

[59] Raatz SK, Golovko MY, Brose SA, et al. Baking reduces prostaglandin, resolvin, and hydroxy-fatty acid content of farm-raised Atlantic salmon (Salmo salar). Journal of Agricultural and Food Chemistry. 2011;**59**:11278-11286

[60] Wang S, Ni L, Fu X, et al. A sulfated polysaccharide from Saccharina japonica suppresses LPS-induced inflammation both in a macrophage cell model via blocking MAPK/NF-κB signal pathways In vitro and a zebrafish model of

embryos and larvae In vivo. Marine Drugs. 2020;**18**:593

[61] Apostolova E, Lukova P, Baldzhieva A, et al. Immunomodulatory and anti-inflammatory effects of fucoidan: A review. Polymers. 2020;**12**:1-25

[62] Mildenberger J, Rebours C. Green (Ulva fenestrata) and Brown (Saccharina latissima) macroalgae similarly modulate inflammatory signaling by activating NF- κ B and dampening IRF in human macrophage-like cells. Journal of Immunology Research. 2024;**2024**(1): 1-14. DOI: 10.1155/2024/8121284

[63] Hervet C, Bussy F, Le Goff C, et al. Marine-sulfated polysaccharides extracts exhibit contrasted time-dependent immunomodulatory and antiviral properties on porcine monocytes and alveolar macrophages. Animals. 2022;**12**:2576

[64] Fang W, Bi D, Zheng R, et al. Identification and activation of TLR4-mediated signalling pathways by alginate-derived guluronate oligosaccharide in RAW264.7 macrophages. Scientific Reports. 2017;**7**:1663

[65] Li Y, Xu Z, Wang J, et al. Alginate-based biomaterial-mediated regulation of macrophages in bone tissue engineering. International Journal of Biological Macromolecules. 2023;**230**:123246

[66] Mo'o FRC, Wilar G, Devkota HP, et al. Ulvan, a polysaccharide from macroalga Ulva sp.: A review of chemistry, biological activities and potential for food and biomedical applications. Applied Sciences. 2020;**10**:5488

[67] Jiang Z, Okimura T, Yamaguchi K, et al. The potent activity of sulfated polysaccharide, ascophyllan, isolated from Ascophyllum nodosum to induce nitric oxide and cytokine production from mouse macrophage RAW264.7 cells: Comparison between ascophyllan and fucoidan. Nitric Oxide. 2011;**25**:407-415

[68] Pei Y, Yang S, Xiao Z, et al. Structural characterization of sulfated polysaccharide isolated from red algae (Gelidium crinale) and antioxidant and anti-inflammatory effects in macrophage cells. Frontiers in Bioengineering and Biotechnology. 2021;**9**:794818. DOI: 10.3389/fbioe.2021.794818

[69] Dai B, Wei D, Zheng NN, et al. Coccomyxa gloeobotrydiformis polysaccharide inhibits lipopolysaccharide-induced inflammation in RAW 264.7 macrophages. Cellular Physiology and Biochemistry. 2019;**51**:2523-2535

[70] Wang Q, Liu W, Yue Y, et al. Proteoglycan from bacillus sp. BS11 inhibits the inflammatory response by suppressing the MAPK and NF-κB pathways in lipopolysaccharide-induced RAW264.7 macrophages. Marine Drugs. 2020;**18**:585

[71] Chotphruethipong L, Chanvorachote P, Reudhabibadh R, et al. Chitooligosaccharide from Pacific white shrimp SHELL chitosan ameliorates inflammation and oxidative stress via NF-κB, Erk1/2, Akt and Nrf2/HO-1 pathways in LPS-induced RAW264.7 macrophage cells. Food. 2023;**12**:2740

[72] Liu M, Li F, Feng S, et al. Evaluation of anticancer and immunomodulatory effects of microwave-extracted polysaccharide from Ruditapes philippinarum. Food. 2024;**13**:3552

[73] Hossain A, Dave D, Shahidi F. Sulfated polysaccharides in sea cucumbers and their biological

properties: A review. International Journal of Biological Macromolecules. 2023;**253**:127329

[74] Goldstein JL, Ho YK, Basu SK, et al. Binding site on macrophages that mediates uptake and degradation of acetylated low density lipoprotein, producing massive cholesterol deposition. Proceedings of the National Academy of Sciences of the United States of America. 1979;**76**:333

[75] Lin Z, Tan X, Zhang Y, et al. Molecular targets and related biologic activities of Fucoidan: A review. Marine Drugs. 2020;**18**:376

[76] Zayed A, Al-Saedi DA, Mensah EO, et al. Fucoidan's molecular targets: A comprehensive review of its unique and multiple targets accounting for promising bioactivities supported by In silico studies. Marine Drugs. 2023;**22**:29

[77] Miyazaki Y, Iwaihara Y, Bak J, et al. The cooperative induction of macrophage activation by fucoidan derived from Cladosiphon okamuranus and β-glucan derived from Saccharomyces cerevisiae. Biochemical and Biophysical Research Communications. 2019;**516**:245-250

[78] Cheng Y, Pan X, Wang J, et al. Fucoidan inhibits NLRP3 inflammasome activation by enhancing p62/SQSTM1-dependent selective autophagy to alleviate atherosclerosis. Oxidative Medicine and Cellular Longevity. 2020;**2020**:3186306

[79] Hou T, Liu X, Zhang S, et al. Anti-inflammatory effects of the Fucoidan from sea cucumber Apostichopus japonicus. Marine Biotechnology (New York, N.Y.). 2025;**27**:32

[80] Li X, Zhu X, Wei Y. Autophagy in atherosclerotic plaque cells: Targeting NLRP3 inflammasome for self-rescue. Biomolecules. 2022;**13**:15

[81] Mihalache CC, Simon HU. Autophagy regulation in macrophages and neutrophils. Experimental Cell Research. 2012;**318**:1187-1192

[82] Huang H, Li X, Zhuang Y, et al. Class A scavenger receptor activation inhibits endoplasmic reticulum stress-induced autophagy in macrophage. Journal of Biomedical Research. 2013;**28**:213

[83] Mirza Z, Al-Saedi DA, Saddeek S, et al. Atheroprotective effect of Fucoidan in THP-1 macrophages by potential upregulation of ABCA1. Biomedicine. 2023;**11**:2929

[84] Li P, Wang H, Shao Q, et al. Fucoidan modulates cytokine production and migration of THP-1-derived macrophages via colony-stimulating factor-1. Molecular Medicine Reports. 2017;**15**:2325-2332

[85] Wang C, Huang L, Huang Y, et al. Study on immunoregulatory effects of Fucoidan from Sargassum graminifolium In vivo and immunoactivation activity of its fecal fermentation products using co-culture model. Molecules. 2023;**28**:7794

[86] Shanura Fernando IP, Kim M, Son KT, et al. Antioxidant activity of marine algal polyphenolic compounds: A mechanistic approach. Journal of Medicinal Food. 2016;**19**:615-628

[87] Nagahawatta DP, Liyanage NM, Jayawardena TU, et al. Marine polyphenols in cardiovascular health: Unraveling structure–activity relationships, mechanisms, and therapeutic implications. International Journal of Molecular Sciences. 2024;**25**:8419

[88] Besednova NN, Andryukov BG, Zaporozhets TS, et al. Molecular targets of brown algae phlorotannins for the

therapy of inflammatory processes of various origins. Marine Drugs. 2022;**20**:243

[89] Catarino MD, Silva A, Cruz MT, et al. Phlorotannins from Fucus vesiculosus: Modulation of inflammatory response by blocking NF-κB signaling pathway. International Journal of Molecular Sciences. 2020;**21**:6897

[90] Yang YI, Jung SH, Lee KT, et al. 8,8′-Bieckol, isolated from edible brown algae, exerts its anti-inflammatory effects through inhibition of NF-κB signaling and ROS production in LPS-stimulated macrophages. International Immunopharmacology. 2014;**23**:460-468

[91] Yang YI, Shin HC, Kim SH, et al. 6,6′-Bieckol, isolated from marine alga Ecklonia cava, suppressed LPS-induced nitric oxide and PGE2 production and inflammatory cytokine expression in macrophages: The inhibition of NFκB. International Immunopharmacology. 2012;**12**:510-517

[92] Sanjeewa KKA, Fernando IPS, Kim HS, et al. Dieckol: An algal polyphenol attenuates urban fine dust-induced inflammation in RAW 264.7 cells via the activation of anti-inflammatory and antioxidant signaling pathways. Journal of Applied Phycology. 2020;**32**:2387-2396

[93] Lee SH, Eom SH, Yoon NY, et al. Fucofuroeckol-A from Eisenia bicyclis inhibits inflammation in lipopolysaccharide-induced mouse macrophages via downregulation of the MAPK/NF-κB signaling pathway. Journal of Chemistry. 2016;**2016**:6509212

[94] Kim KC, Kang KA, Zhang R, et al. Up-regulation of Nrf2-mediated heme oxygenase-1 expression by eckol, a phlorotannin compound, through activation of Erk and PI3K/Akt. International Journal of Biochemistry and Cell Biology. 2010;**42**:297-305

[95] Shibata T, Nagayama K, Tanaka R, et al. Inhibitory effects of brown algal phlorotannins on secretory phospholipase A2s, lipoxygenases and cyclooxygenases. Journal of Applied Phycology. 2003;**15**:61-66

[96] Kurihara H, Konno R, Takahashi K, Fucophlorethol C. A phlorotannin as a lipoxygenase inhibitor. Bioscience, Biotechnology, and Biochemistry. 2015;**79**:1954-1956

[97] Kim MJ, Lee HH, Jeong JW, et al. Anti-inflammatory effects of 5-hydroxy-3,6,7,8,3′,′4-hexamethoxyflavone via NF-κB inactivation in lipopolysaccharide-stimulated RAW 264.7 macrophage. Molecular Medicine Reports. 2014;**9**:1197-1203

[98] Chen J, Liu H, Fu Y, et al. Kaempferol attenuates macrophage M1 polarization and liver fibrosis by inhibiting mitogen-activated protein kinase/nuclear factor κB signaling pathway. The Journal of Pharmacology and Experimental Therapeutics. 2025;**392**:103533

[99] Tsai C-F, Chen G-W, Chen Y-C, et al. Regulatory effects of quercetin on M1/M2 macrophage polarization and oxidative/antioxidative balance. Nutrients. 2021;**14**:67

[100] Choi YK, Ye B-R, Kim E-A, et al. Bis (3-bromo-4,5-dihydroxybenzyl) ether, a novel bromophenol from the marine red alga Polysiphonia morrowii that suppresses LPS-induced inflammatory response by inhibiting ROS-mediated ERK signaling pathway in RAW 264.7 macrophages. Biomedicine and Pharmacotherapy. 2018;**103**:1170-1177

[101] Kang NJ, Han SC, Kang HJ, et al. Anti-inflammatory effect of

3-bromo-4,5-dihydroxybenzaldehyde, a component of Polysiphonia morrowii, in vivo and in vitro. Toxicology Research. 2017;**33**:325-332

[102] Wang R, Zhu W, Peng J, et al. Lipid rafts as potential mechanistic targets underlying the pleiotropic actions of polyphenols. Critical Reviews in Food Science and Nutrition. 2021;**62**:311-324

[103] Liu M, Li W, Chen Y, et al. Fucoxanthin: A promising compound for human inflammation-related diseases. Life Sciences. 2020;**255**:117850. DOI: 10.1016/j.lfs.2020.117850

[104] Zhang L, Wang H, Fan Y, et al. Fucoxanthin provides neuroprotection in models of traumatic brain injury via the Nrf2-ARE and Nrf2-autophagy pathways. Scientific Reports. 2017;**7**:1-15

[105] Mao H, Wang L, Xiong Y, et al. Fucoxanthin attenuates oxidative damage by activating the Sirt1/Nrf2/HO-1 signaling pathway to protect the kidney from ischemia-reperfusion injury. Oxidative Medicine and Cellular Longevity. 2022;**2022**:7444430

[106] Lee N, Youn K, Yoon JH, et al. The role of fucoxanthin as a potent Nrf2 activator via Akt/GSK-3β/Fyn Axis against amyloid-β peptide-induced oxidative damage. Antioxidants. 2023;**12**:629

[107] Kim MB, Kang H, Li Y, et al. Fucoxanthin inhibits lipopolysaccharide-induced inflammation and oxidative stress by activating nuclear factor E2-related factor 2 via the phosphatidylinositol 3-kinase/AKT pathway in macrophages. European Journal of Nutrition. 2021;**60**:3315-3324

[108] Wu W, Han H, Liu J, et al. Fucoxanthin prevents 6-OHDA-induced neurotoxicity by targeting Keap1. Oxidative Medicine and Cellular Longevity. 2021;**2021**:6688708

[109] Ding YW, Zhao GJ, Li XL, et al. SIRT1 exerts protective effects against paraquat-inducedinjury in mouse type II alveolar epithelial cellsby deacetylating NRF2 in vitro. International Journal of Molecular Medicine. 2016;**37**:1049-1058

[110] Lee A-H, Shin H-Y, Park J-H, et al. Fucoxanthin from microalgae Phaeodactylum tricornutum inhibits pro-inflammatory cytokines by regulating both NF-κB and NLRP3 inflammasome activation. Scientific Reports. 2021;**11**:543

[111] Jin W, Yang L, Yi Z, et al. Anti-inflammatory effects of fucoxanthinol in LPS-induced RAW264.7 cells through the NAAA-PEA pathway. Marine Drugs. 2020;**18**:222

[112] Jinendiran S, Dahms HU, Dileep Kumar BS, et al. Diapolycopenedioic-acid-diglucosyl ester and keto-myxocoxanthin glucoside ester: Novel carotenoids derived from Exiguobacterium acetylicum S01 and evaluation of their anticancer and anti-inflammatory activities. Bioorganic Chemistry. 2020;**103**:104149

[113] Hadad N, Levy R. The synergistic anti-inflammatory effects of lycopene, lutein, β-carotene, and carnosic acid combinations via redox-based inhibition of NF-κB signaling. Free Radical Biology and Medicine. 2012;**53**:1381-1391

[114] Tounsi L, Ben Hlima H, Hentati F, et al. Microalgae: A promising source of bioactive phycobiliproteins. Marine Drugs. 2023;**21**:440

[115] Lee D, Nishizawa M, Shimizu Y, et al. Anti-inflammatory effects of dulse (Palmaria palmata) resulting from the simultaneous water-extraction

of phycobiliproteins and chlorophyll a. Food Research International. 2017;**100**:514-521

[116] Chang MX, Xiong F. Astaxanthin and its effects in inflammatory responses and inflammation-associated diseases: Recent advances and future directions. Molecules. 2020;**25**:5342

[117] Zhou X, Zhang J, Li Y, et al. Astaxanthin inhibits microglia M1 activation against inflammatory injury triggered by lipopolysaccharide through down-regulating miR-31-5p. Life Sciences. 2021;**267**:118943

[118] Zhang XS, Lu Y, Li W, et al. Astaxanthin ameliorates oxidative stress and neuronal apoptosis via SIRT1/NRF2/Prx2/ASK1/p38 after traumatic brain injury in mice. British Journal of Pharmacology. 2021;**178**:1114-1132

[119] Jin M, Chen X, Zheng L, et al. Astaxanthin-loaded polylactic acid-glycolic acid nanoparticles alleviates atherosclerosis by suppressing macrophage ferroptosis via the NRF2/SLC7A11/GPX4 pathway. Archives of Biochemistry and Biophysics. 2025;**765**:110316

[120] Liu A, Li R, Zaaboul F, et al. Proteomic analysis reveals the mechanisms of the astaxanthin suppressed foam cell formation. Life Sciences. 2023;**325**:121774

[121] Zhang Z, Qiu Y, Li W, et al. Astaxanthin alleviates foam cell formation and promotes cholesterol efflux in ox-LDL-induced RAW264.7 cells via CircTPP2/miR-3073b-5p/ABCA1 pathway. Molecules. 2023;**28**:1701

[122] Inoue M, Tanabe H, Matsumoto A, et al. Astaxanthin functions differently as a selective peroxisome proliferator-activated receptor γ modulator in adipocytes and macrophages. Biochemical Pharmacology. 2012;**84**:692-700

[123] Zhou J, Liu W, Zhao X, et al. Natural melanin/alginate hydrogels achieve cardiac repair through ROS scavenging and macrophage polarization. Advanced Science. 2021;**8**(20):2100505. DOI: 10.1002/advs.202100505

[124] Guryanova SV, Balandin SV, Belogurova-Ovchinnikova OY, et al. Marine invertebrate antimicrobial peptides and their potential as novel peptide antibiotics. Marine Drugs. 2023;**21**:503

[125] Han H, Teng D, Mao R, et al. Marine peptide-N6NH2 and its derivative-GUON6NH2 have potent antimicrobial activity against intracellular Edwardsiella tarda in vitro and in vivo. Frontiers in Microbiology. 2021;**12**:637427. DOI: 10.3389/fmicb.2021.637427

[126] Li T, Wang Z, Han H, et al. Potent intracellular antibacterial activity of a marine peptide-N6NH2 and its D-enantiomer against multidrug-resistant Aeromonas veronii. Applied Microbiology and Biotechnology. 2021;**105**:2351-2361

[127] Li Z, Wang X, Teng D, et al. Improved antibacterial activity of a marine peptide-N2 against intracellular salmonella typhimurium by conjugating with cell-penetrating peptides-bLFcin6/Tat11. European Journal of Medicinal Chemistry. 2018;**145**:263-272

[128] Chen J, Nie L, Chen J. Mudskipper (Boleophthalmus pectinirostris) Hepcidin-1 and Hepcidin-2 present different gene expression profile and antibacterial activity and possess distinct protective effect against Edwardsiella tarda infection. Probiotics and Antimicrobial Proteins. 2018;**10**:176-185

[129] Hsieh C, Rajanbabu V, Pan C-Y, et al. Transcriptome analysis reveals modulation of differentially expressed genes in LPS-treated mouse macrophages (RAW264.7 cells) by grouper (Epinephelus coioides) Epinecidin-1. Fish and Shellfish Immunology. 2023;**139**:108880

[130] Vilasi A, Monti MC, Tosco A, et al. Differential in gel electrophoresis (DIGE) comparative proteomic analysis of macrophages cell cultures in response to Perthamide C treatment. Marine Drugs. 2013;**11**:1288

[131] Li Y, Li J, Lin SJ, et al. Preparation of antioxidant peptide by microwave-assisted hydrolysis of collagen and its protective effect against H2O2-induced damage of RAW264.7 cells. Marine Drugs. 2019;**17**:642

[132] Qian B, Zhao X, Yang Y, et al. Antioxidant and anti-inflammatory peptide fraction from oyster soft tissue by enzymatic hydrolysis. Food Science and Nutrition. 2020;**8**:3947-3956

[133] Saisavoey T, Sangtanoo P, Reamtong O, et al. Free radical scavenging and anti-inflammatory potential of a protein hydrolysate derived from salmon bones on RAW 264.7 macrophage cells. Journal of the Science of Food and Agriculture. 2019;**99**:5112-5121

[134] Kim YS, Ahn CB, Je JY. Anti-inflammatory action of high molecular weight Mytilus edulis hydrolysates fraction in LPS-induced RAW264.7 macrophage via NF-κB and MAPK pathways. Food Chemistry. 2016;**202**:9-14

[135] Cian RE, López-Posadas R, Drago SR, et al. A Porphyra columbina hydrolysate upregulates IL-10 production in rat macrophages and lymphocytes through an NF-κB, and p38 and JNK dependent mechanism. Food Chemistry. 2012;**134**:1982-1990

[136] Lin H, Li W, Sun R, et al. Purification and characterization of a novel immunoregulatory peptide from Sipunculus nudus L. protein. Food Science and Nutrition. 2023;**11**:7779

[137] Marasinghe CK, Yoon S, Je J. Two peptides LLRLTDL and GYALPCDCL inhibit foam cell formation through activating PPARγ/LXR-α signaling pathway in oxLDL-treated RAW264.7 macrophages. BioFactors. 2024;**50**:1161-1175

[138] Kim E-N, Gao M, Choi H, et al. Marine microorganism-derived macrolactins inhibit inflammatory mediator effects in LPS-induced macrophage and microglial cells by regulating BACH1 and HO-1/Nrf2 signals through inhibition of TLR4 activation. Molecules. 2020;**25**:656

[139] Yang Y, Wang J, Tian Y, et al. Equisetin protects from atherosclerosis in vivo by binding to STAT3 and inhibiting its activity. Pharmacological Research. 2024;**206**:107289

[140] Fu J, Luo X, Lin M, et al. Marine-fungi-derived gliotoxin promotes autophagy to suppress mycobacteria tuberculosis infection in macrophage. Marine Drugs. 2023;**21**:616

[141] Keeler DM, Grandal MK, McCall JR. Brevenal, a marine natural product, is anti-inflammatory and an immunomodulator of macrophage and lung epithelial cells. Marine Drugs. 2019;**17**:184

[142] Jayawardena TU, Sanjeewa KKA, Lee HG, et al. Particulate matter-induced inflammation/oxidative stress in macrophages: Fucosterol from Padina

boryana as a potent protector, activated via NF-κB/MAPK pathways and Nrf2/HO-1 involvement. Marine Drugs. 2020;**18**:628

[143] Germano G, Frapolli R, Belgiovine C, et al. Role of macrophage targeting in the antitumor activity of trabectedin. Cancer Cell. 2013;**23**:249-262

[144] Škrovánková S. Seaweed vitamins as nutraceuticals. Advances in Food and Nutrition Research. 2011;**64**:357-369

[145] Udaypal GRK, Mehariya S, et al. Microalgae-derived tocopherols: Biotechnological advances in production and its therapeutic potentials. Sustainable Chemistry and Pharmacy. 2024;**42**:101791

[146] Lee GY, Han SN. The role of vitamin E in immunity. Nutrients. 2018;**10**:1614

[147] Jamalvandi M, Khayyatzadeh SS, Hayati MJ, et al. The role of fat-soluble vitamins in efferocytosis. Cell Biochemistry and Function. 2024;**42**(2):e3972. DOI: 10.1002/cbf.3972

[148] Holick MF. Vitamin D: A millenium perspective. Journal of Cellular Biochemistry. 2003;**88**:296-307

[149] Bikle DD, Vitamin D. Regulation of immune function. Current Osteoporosis Reports. 2022;**20**:186

[150] Furman D, Campisi J, Verdin E, et al. Chronic inflammation in the etiology of disease across the life span. Nature Medicine. 2019;**25**:1822

[151] Monteleone G, Moscardelli A, Colella A, et al. Immune-mediated inflammatory diseases: Common and different pathogenic and clinical features. Autoimmunity Reviews. 2023;**22**:103410

[152] Leyane TS, Jere SW, Houreld NN. Oxidative stress in ageing and chronic degenerative pathologies: Molecular mechanisms involved in counteracting oxidative stress and chronic inflammation. International Journal of Molecular Sciences. 2022;**23**:7273

[153] Yu X, Pu H, Voss M. Overview of anti-inflammatory diets and their promising effects on non-communicable diseases. The British Journal of Nutrition. 2024;**132**:898